Visceral Pain

Visceral Pain

Clinical, pathophysiological and therapeutic aspects

Edited by

Maria Adele Giamberardino

Associate Professor of Internal Medicine,
Department of Medicine and Science of Ageing,
"G. D'Annunzio" University of Chieti, Italy

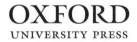

OXFORD
UNIVERSITY PRESS

OXFORD
UNIVERSITY PRESS

Great Clarendon Street, Oxford OX2 6DP

Oxford University Press is a department of the University of Oxford.
It furthers the University's objective of excellence in research, scholarship,
and education by publishing worldwide in

Oxford New York

Auckland Cape Town Dar es Salaam Hong Kong Karachi
Kuala Lumpur Madrid Melbourne Mexico City Nairobi
New Delhi Shanghai Taipei Toronto

With offices in

Argentina Austria Brazil Chile Czech Republic France Greece
Guatemala Hungary Italy Japan Poland Portugal Singapore
South Korea Switzerland Thailand Turkey Ukraine Vietnam

Oxford is a registered trade mark of Oxford University Press
in the UK and in certain other countries

Published in the United States
by Oxford University Press Inc., New York

British Library Cataloguing in Publication Data

Data available

Library of Congress Cataloging in Publication Data

Data available

Typeset by Newgen Imaging Systems (P) Ltd., Chennai, India
Printed in Great Britain
on acid-free paper by
Ashford Colour Press Ltd, Gosport, Hants.

ISBN 978-0-19-923519-3

10 9 8 7 6 5 4 3 2 1

Contents

Preface

Visceral pain is a major clinical problem and the reason for a vast proportion of patients' requests for medical consultation. Community surveys reveal, for example, that over 25% of people complain of intermittent abdominal pain, 20% have chest pain and 24% of women suffer from recurrent/chronic pelvic pain. Many painful conditions from internal organs are, in addition, potentially life threatening, as in the case of myocardial and intestinal infarction or acute pancreatitis. Prompt recognition of visceral pain is thus mandatory in current medical practice, but is not an easy task as its characteristics are often atypical and variable in time. The interpretation is further complicated when the same patient has concurrent painful conditions in more than one internal organ, showing an intricate and often misleading complex of symptoms. Furthermore, in spite of its clinical impact, pain from internal organs is still incompletely understood in its mechanisms, which impacts negatively on therapy.

It is clear that a thorough knowledge of the different expressions of visceral pain is crucial for the clinician to make a correct diagnosis, whereas and an up-to-date awareness of progress in research on pathophysiology is of great help in orientating towards the best targeted therapy. While most books on visceral pain are extensive treatises, useful for in depth study of specific aspects of the topic, this "Visceral Pain" pocketbook is conceived to provide synthetic - though complete - readily-available information for interpretation and treatment of the symptom in current medical practice. This publication, by allowing rapid consultation, is primarily aimed at helping health care professionals in their practical approach to the visceral pain patient - in primary care, internal medicine specialties and pain management - but we trust it will also be of interest to basic scientists in physiology, pharmacology and neurosciences, as well as informative for students in medical, nursing or pharmacy disciplines. The first part is a general section addressing the epidemiology and characteristics of the major visceral pain phenomena, the fundamentals of their neurophysiological mechanisms and the principles of treatment. The second part consists of chapters providing diagnostic and therapeutic guidelines for the most important diseases that cause visceral pain from different apparati and body districts. The authors of 'Visceral Pain' are worldwide specialists in their fields, from both clinical and basic science backgrounds. I am deeply grateful to all of them for providing such valuable scientific contributions; thanks to their efforts, I hope this booklet will not only help the readers to answer practical medical queries but also stimulate further their professional interest in the fascinating field of visceral pain.

Maria Adele Giamberardino

Contributors

Lars Arendt-Nielsen
Center for Sensory-Motor
Interactions
Department of Health Science
and Technology
Aalborg University
Denmark

Qasim Aziz
Wingate Institute of
Neurogastroenterology
London, UK

Andrew Paul Baranowski
University College London
Hospitals NHS Foundation Trust
The National Hospital for
Neurology and Neurosurgery
Queen Square, London, UK

Karen J. Berkley
Program in Neuroscience
Florida State University
Tallahassee, Florida, USA

Mats Börjesson
Associate Professor
Sahlgrenska University
Hospital/Östra
Göteborg, Sweden

Fernando Cervero
Anaesthesia Research Unit
McGill Centre for Research on Pain
McGill University
Montreal, Canada

Raffaele Costantini
Department of General and
Laparoscopic Surgery
"G. D'Annunzio" University of Chieti
Italy

Asbjörn Mohr Drewes
Center for Visceral Biomechanics
and Pain
Department of Gastroenterology
Aalborg University Hospital
Denmark

Maria Adele Giamberardino
Department of Medicine and
Science of Aging
"G. D'Annunzio" University of Chieti
Italy

Smita L.S. Halder
Department of GI Sciences
University of Manchester, UK

Peter Holzer
Research Unit of Translational
Neurogastroenterology
Institute of Experimental and
Clinical Pharmacology
Medical University of Graz
Graz, Austria

Ulrike Holzer-Petsche
Research Unit of Translational
Neurogastroenterology
Institute of Experimental and
Clinical Pharmacology
Medical University of Graz
Graz, Austria

Jennifer M.A. Laird
AstraZeneca R& D Montreal and
Department of Pharmacology
and Therapeutics
McGill Centre for Research on Pain
McGill University, Monteal
Canada

G. Richard Locke III
Enteric Neuroscience Program
Division of Gastroenterology
Mayo Clinic College of Medicine
Rochester, USA

Sebastiano Mercadante
Palliative Medicine
University of Palermo
Anesthesia and Intensive Care Unit
& Pain Relief and Palliative Care Unit
La Maddalena Cancer Center
Palermo, Italy

Lukas Van Oudenhove
Department of Neurosciences
Division of Psychiatry
University of Leuven
University Hospital Gasthuisberg
Belgium

Pamela Stratton
Reproductive Biology and
Medicine Branch
National Institute of Child Health and
Development
National Institutes of Health
Bethesda, USA

Abbreviations

ACC	Anterior Cingulate Cortex
AMPA	Alpha-amino-3-hydroxy-5-methyl-4-isoxazolepropionic acid
BGA	Brain-Gut Axis
CABG	Coronary Artery Bypass Grafting
CAD	Coronary Artery Disease
CBT	Cognitive Behavioural Therapy
CCK	Cholecystokinin
CCU	Coronary Care Unit
CGRP	Calcitonin Gene-Related Peptide
CNS	Central Nervous System
COMT	Catechol-O-Methyl-Transferase
CRD	Colo-Rectal Distension
CRF	Corticotropin-Releasing Factor
CS	Central Sensitization
EAU CPPGG	European Association for Urology, Chronic Pelvic Pain, Guidelines Group
EMS	Emotional Motor System
ENDO	Surgically-induced endometrial cysts
ESSIC	European Association for the Study of Bladder Pain Syndrome/Interstitial Cystitis
FAPSynd	Functional Abdominal Pain Syndrome
FD	Functional Dyspepsia
FGID	Functional Gastrointestinal Disorders
GORD	Gastroesophageal Reflux Disease
GI	Gastrointestinal
GnRH	Gonadotrophin-Releasing Hormone
IBD	Inflammatory Bowel Disease
IBS	Irritable Bowel Syndrome
LC	Locus Coeruleus
NCCP	Non-cardiac Chest Pain
NCPB	Neurolytic Coeliac Plexus Block
NE	Nutcracker oesophagus

NERD	Non-Erosive Gastroesophageal Reflux Disease
NHS	National Healthcare System
NMDA	N-methyl-D-aspartate
NRS	Numerical Rating Scale
NSAIDS	Non-Steroidal Anti-Inflammatory Drugs
NTS	Nucleus of the Solitary Tract
PAG	Periaqueductal Grey
PARs	Protease-Activated Receptors
PFC	Prefrontal Cortex
PGs	Prostaglandins
PMM	Punctate Midline Myelotomy
PPI	Proton Pump Inhibitors
PS	Peripheral Sensitization
PTEN	Phosphatase and Tensin homolog, (deleted on chromosome Ten)
RANTES	Regulated upon Activation, Normal T-cell Expressed, and Secreted
RAP	Recurrent Abdominal Pain
SNRIs	Selective Noradrenaline and Serotonin Reuptake Inhibitors
SSRIs	Selective Serotonin Reuptake Inhibitors
TCAs	Tricyclic Antidepressants
TRP	Transient Receptor Potential
VAS	Visual Analogue Scale
VRS	Verbal Rating Scale

Chapter 1

Epidemiology and social impact of visceral pain

Smita L.S. Halder and G. Richard Locke III

Key points

- Visceral pain can arise from the chest, abdomen or pelvis and is a common symptom in the population
- The majority of pain is indeterminate and thought to be functional in origin, but its psychosocial impact on a sufferer may be considerable
- Visceral pain disorders place a large economic burden on healthcare resources and on the workplace through lost productivity.

1.1 Introduction

Chronic and recurrent pain affecting the chest, abdomen, or pelvic region is experienced by a large number of people in the community. Surveys have shown prevalence rates among adults of 25% for intermittent abdominal pain and 20% for chest pain; 24% of women suffer from pelvic pain at any time point. For over two-thirds of sufferers, pain is accepted as part of daily life and symptoms are self-managed; a small proportion defer to specialists for help. The minority that seeks care is different from those who do not, and thus population-based studies are needed to truly understand the epidemiology of these visceral pain syndromes. Visceral pain conditions are associated with diminished quality of life, and exert a huge cost burden through medical expenses and lost productivity in the workplace. This review will outline the epidemiology and social impact of the most common visceral pain syndromes.

1.2 Abdominal pain

Abdominal pain can be an indication of specific underlying disease, but in many sufferers, all diagnostic tests are either normal or negative. Such pain is thought to be visceral in origin as most often it has an indistinct, crampy character and is poorly localized. Surgeons refer to it as non-specific abdominal pain, older textbooks comment on non-organic pain, and pain in children is known as recurrent abdominal pain (RAP). Some use the term chronic functional abdominal pain syndrome, but this is primarily a diagnosis for people with the most severe pain being seen in academic health centers. In the community many people simply have abdominal pain.

1.2.1 Epidemiology of abdominal pain

Abdominal pain is common in the community with prevalence rates between 22% and 28%. Women are more likely to report pain than men. About one in five of people in the community with abdominal pain consult a physician. In contrast, the majority of respondents complain of impairment in carrying out usual activities due to the pain, with the level of impairment similar between the sexes. This implies that abdominal pain impacts upon the daily lives of a vast number of people in whom no formal diagnosis is made.

The natural history of abdominal pain in the adult population is largely unknown. Abdominal symptoms have been observed to relapse and remit over the course of a year. The overall prevalence rate remains constant, but this is accounted for by considerable symptom turnover. The onset rate is about 10% and the disappearance rate is 35%. Prevalence rates are stable because the absolute numbers of people with onset and disappearance are matched.

1.2.2 Burden of abdominal pain on health care

Functional abdominal pain makes up a major component of the clinical spectrum of hospital admissions for abdominal pain. This is not a new problem. In 1966, abdominal pain for which no definite explanation could be found was the tenth most common cause of admission to hospital for any reason in men and the sixth most common cause in women. Of those who were admitted with undiagnosed abdominal pain, there was a higher preponderance of young females, and there was a significant excess of people with a previous admission for psychiatric reasons. The situation has not changed to the present day. Up to 67% of consecutive admissions to a teaching hospital surgical ward are for 'non-specific' abdominal pain. In Britain, the mean cost to the NHS per patient was estimated at £807, which was mainly attributed to the in-patient stay. Extrapolating to the whole of the UK, the economic burden of non-specific abdominal pain was postulated to be in excess of £100 million per year.

1.3 Specific visceral and abdominal pain syndromes

1.3.1 Irritable Bowel Syndrome

The irritable bowel syndrome (IBS) is a chronic gastrointestinal disorder characterized by recurrent abdominal pain that is associated with defecation. The symptoms do not have a structural or biochemical explanation. Many population-based surveys around the globe have assessed the individual symptoms of irritable bowel syndrome and estimated the prevalence to be between 8% and 22%. The prevalence of IBS is higher in women and lower in the elderly.

Data regarding incidence are much more difficult to obtain. Information on symptom onset and disappearance can be obtained by repeated surveys over time. Roughly 10% of the general population will report the onset of IBS symptoms over a one-year period. Approximately one-third of people with IBS symptoms will report symptom resolution over time. The incidence of a clinical diagnosis of IBS has been estimated to be 196 to 260 per 100,000 person years. This is not the true incidence of IBS but rather the rate at which the diagnosis of IBS is made in the clinic. These numbers may seem low; however, when multiplied by 30 years of disease duration and then doubled to reflect the rate of those seeking health care, the result is 12%, which matches the prevalence reported in the symptom surveys. Of note, these incidence rates are also much higher than the rates reported for colorectal cancer and inflammatory bowel disease (IBD) which are 50 and 10 per 100,000 person years, respectively.

The cost of IBS is high in terms of health care utilization (outpatient costs, hospitalization costs, prescription costs) and employer costs. IBS accounts for 25–50% of referrals to gastroenterologists, 96,000 hospital discharges, 3 million physician visits, and 2.2 million prescriptions annually. Although only 9% of people with IBS symptoms in the community seek care annually, these people miss more days from work and have more physician visits for both gastrointestinal and non-gastrointestinal complaints than the general population. By one estimate, people with IBS incur an extra $313 per person per year in charges compared with controls. If extrapolated to the U.S. population, the resulting cost of IBS is $8 billion per year.

Numerous studies have shown that the quality of life of individuals with IBS is lower than the general population and even lower than individuals with congestive heart failure. Many patients with IBS have multiple non-gastrointestinal symptoms (e.g., fatigue, musculoskeletal pain), and while this association is unexplained, it can confound epidemiological association studies.

1.3.2 **Chronic Functional Abdominal Pain Syndrome**

Functional Abdominal Pain Syndrome (FAPSynd) is defined as 'pain for at least six months that is poorly related to gut function and is associated with some loss of daily activities.' In FAPSynd, there is no disordered bowel motility and thus bowel disruption is not a prominent feature. Pain is only judged functional once an organic reason can be safely excluded and is considered to exist in the absence of structural or biochemical abnormalities.

FAPSynd, in its strictest form, is relatively infrequent in the general population. In one study, FAPSynd was seen in 2% of the respondents. Despite the low prevalence, the socioeconomic impact of FAPSynd was immense with sufferers missing three times as many work-days in the previous year compared to those without abdominal symptoms. Patients who are referred to gastroenterologists have further cost implications as they undergo numerous diagnostic procedures and treatments and make a disproportionate number of health care visits.

1.3.3 **Non-cardiac chest pain/functional chest pain**

Chest pain is an alarm symptom that brings hundreds of thousands of people to seek health care worldwide each year. In the population, 28% of people report experiencing some form of chest pain in the past year. Due to the high prevalence and serious morbidity of coronary artery disease, the complaint of chest pain is treated as cardiac in origin until proven otherwise. Still, 10–20% of patients admitted to a coronary care unit are shown to have an esophageal disease. The challenge for health care providers has been differentiating those with acute coronary syndromes from those with other causes for chest pain.

Noncardiac chest pain (NCCP) is defined by the absence of significant stenoses in the major epicardial coronary arteries. Each year about 450,000 people with chest pain have normal coronary angiograms. Despite how many suffer from NCCP, little is known about the epidemiology or natural history of chest pain in the community. Moreover, little population-based data has been published to date that help characterize NCCP in the community. The prevalence of NCCP has been estimated to be 23% based on self-report only. The prevalence in the community is similar by gender but a higher female-to-male ratio is seen in tertiary care referral centers. It has been observed that there is significant overlap with NCCP and frequent gastroesophageal reflux symptoms.

1.3.4 **Anorectal pain (proctalgia)**

Proctalgia can be associated with organic or functional disorders; the two most common functional disorders are levator ani syndrome and proctalgia fugax. The main differences between them are the nature and duration of pain. The pain of levator ani syndrome is described as a dull ache or pressure-like discomfort, which can last for hours. The estimated prevalence of levator ani syndrome lies between 7–11.3%, with a higher rate seen in females and those less than 45 years of age.

Proctalgia fugax is characterized by sudden and severe shooting pain in the rectal area which lasts for seconds to minutes and then disappears completely until the next episode. This syndrome is more common than levator ani, with 14% of those questioned in a population survey reporting at least one episode and 5% reporting at least six episodes yearly.

1.3.5 **Recurrent abdominal pain in children**

Abdominal pain is a part of life of the average child, with 12-month period prevalence rates varying from 20% in a population sample to 44% in a General Practice cohort. In up to one-fifth of affected children, episodes are recurrent and interspersed by symptom-free periods and this is termed recurrent abdominal pain (RAP). In the majority of children, the abdominal pain is vague and typically situated in the peri-umbilical area. Physical examination is strikingly normal and laboratory investigations unremarkable. As an organic diagnosis is made in less than 10% of cases, this has led to the long-held belief that most childhood abdominal pain is functional in origin. Studies dating back to the 1950s have reported that 10% of children aged 5–14 years suffered from RAP. Subsequent published prevalence rates have varied between 9% to nearly 25%. Whether there is a sex difference in the prevalence rates is disputed, but it is generally acknowledged that as children get older, incidence rates are higher in girls than boys. In the late adolescent years, there is a sharp decline in incidence.

In many ways, the burden of illness is similar to adult unexplained abdominal pain. Only 30% of emergency hospital visits for abdominal pain result in a definitive diagnosis, and in up to one-third of emergency appendectomies performed for abdominal pain, the appendix is normal. The financial impact of abdominal pain is overshadowed by the effects on the child. Many school days are lost through recurrent clinic visits or hospitalizations which, in addition to the disruption of social activities, may be detrimental to the child's well-being and development.

1.3.6 Pelvic pain

Chronic pelvic pain is characterized by lower abdominal pain that could be related to a multitude of underlying causes. It tends to affect women but the true definition excludes pain related to pregnancy, menstruation or malignancy. Community studies have estimated the prevalence rate to be around 24%. Prevalence rates vary with age with increasing rates found in older women. There are also racial differences; in the UK, Caucasian women report higher rates of pain compared to non-Caucasian women.

A high proportion do not seek medical help for their symptoms, but those who do tend to have more severe pain, nearly all use medications to alleviate symptoms, and the majority report an adverse impact on their daily life. There are higher rates of depression, somatisation and a history of abuse in clinic attenders with pelvic pain than the general population.

Incidence rates in the community are estimated at 1.6/1000 women at risk (age 18–50 years) per month, which translates to 1.9% per year. Pelvic pain symptoms are chronic with a third of women having persistent symptoms after 2 years.

Chronic pelvic Pain exerts a high economic burden on the healthcare system. A hospital-based UK study estimated the direct treatment costs at £158 million, with indirect costs of £24 million. In the US population, direct costs can reach almost $1 billion and indirect costs due to work absences are estimated at $500 million. Almost three-quarters of affected women do not seek medical attention for their symptoms, but the economic burden of this disorder on society is still significant.

1.4 **Conclusions**

This chapter has reviewed the epidemiology of the most common visceral pain disorders. Although many of these people have not had diagnostic testing to exclude organic diseases, the current literature suggests that most of these people have functional problems. In this difficult to manage group of subjects, an understanding of the mechanisms causing symptoms will be a step towards alleviating the suffering and economic costs incurred.

Key References

Chang L, Toner BB, Fukudo S, Guthrie E, Locke GR, Norton NJ, et al. (2006). Gender, age, society, culture, and the patient's perspective in the functional gastrointestinal disorders. *Gastroenterology*. **130**(5): 1435–36.

Drossman DA, Li Z, Andruzzi E, Temple RD, Talley NJ, Thompson WG, et al. (1993). U.S. householder survey of functional gastrointestinal disorders. Prevalence, socio-demography, and health impact. *Dig Dis Sci*. **38**(9): 1569–80.

El-Serag H, Olden K, Bjorkman D (2002). Health-related quality of life among persons with irritable bowel syndrome: a systematic review. *Aliment Pharmacol Ther*. **16**(6): 1171–85.

Goodacre S, Cross E, Arnold J, Angelini K, Capewell S, Nicholl J (2005). The health care burden of acute chest pain. *Heart*. **91**(2): 229–30.

Grace VM, Zondervan KT (2004). Chronic pelvic pain in New Zealand: prevalence, pain severity, diagnoses and use of the health services. *Aust N Z J Public Health*. **28**(4): 369–75.

Halder S, Locke GR, Schleck CD, Zinsmeister AR, Melton LJ, Talley NJ (2007). Natural history of functional gastrointestinal disorders: A 12-year longitudinal population-based study. *Gastroenterology*. **133**(3): 799–807.

Hotopf M, Carr S, Mayou R, Wadsworth M, Wessely S (1998). Why do children have chronic abdominal pain, and what happens to them when they grow up? Population based cohort study. *BMJ*. **316**(7139): 1196–200.

Ockene IS, Shay MJ, Alpert JS, Weiner BH, Dalen JE (1980). Unexplained chest pain in patients with normal coronary arteriograms: a follow-up study of functional status. *N Engl J Med*. **303**(22): 1249–52.

Sandler RS, Everhart JE, Donowitz M, Adams E, Cronin K, Goodman C, et al. (2002). The burden of selected digestive diseases in the United States. *Gastroenterology*. **122**(5): 1500–11.

Sandler RS, Stewart WF, Liberman JN, Ricci JA, Zorich NL (2000). Abdominal pain, bloating, and diarrhea in the United States: prevalence and impact. *Dig Dis Sci*. **45**(6): 1166–71.

Stones RW, Selfe SA, Fransman S, Horn SA (2000). Psychosocial and economic impact of chronic pelvic pain. *Baillieres Best Pract Res Clin Obstet Gynaecol*. **14**(3): 415–31.

Talley N, Zinsmeister AR Melton LJ 3rd (1995). Irritable bowel syndrome in a community: symptom subgroups, risk factors and health care utilization. *Am J Epidemiol*. **142**(1): 76–83.

Talley NJ, Gabriel SE, Harmsen WS, Zinsmeister AR, Evans RW (1995). Medical costs in community subjects with irritable bowel syndrome. *Gastroenterology*. **109**(6): 1736–41.

Talley NJ, O'Keefe EA, Zinsmeister AR, Melton LJ 3rd (1992). Prevalence of gastro-intestinal symptoms in the elderly: a population-based study. *Gastroenterology*. **102**(3): 895–901.

Thompson WG (1981). Proctalgia fugax. *Dig Dis Sci*. **26**(12): 1121–4.

Scharff L (1997). Recurrent abdominal pain in children: a review of psychological factors and treatment. *Clin Psychol Rev*. **17**(2): 145–66.

Zondervan KT, Yudkin PL, Vessey MP, Jenkinson CP, Dawes MG, Barlow DH, *et al.* (2001). The community prevalence of chronic pelvic pain in women and associated illness behaviour. *Br J Gen Pract*. **51**(468): 541–7.

8

Chapter 2

Visceral pain phenomena in the clinical setting and their interpretation

Maria Adele Giamberardino and Raffaele Costantini

> ## Key points
>
> - Visceral pain presentation in the clinic depends on the temporal evolution of the painful process: true visceral pain, referred pain without and with hyperalgesia. It also depends on the nature and location of the primary insult: visceral hyperalgesia, viscero-visceral hyperalgesia
> - True visceral pain occurs at an early stage: it is midline, poorly defined, associated with marked neurovegetative signs and emotional reactions, but not with local hypersensitivity. Its features mostly depend on the low density of innervation of viscera and strong functional divergence of visceral input in the central nervous system
> - Referred pain replaces true visceral pain after minutes or hours. It is felt in the somatic area neuromerically connected to the affected organ, is sharper and better defined and accompanied by mild neurovegetative signs. At the beginning it is not associated with local somatic tissue hypersensitivity (referred pain without hyperalgesia – R1); subsequently hypersensitivity occurs (referred pain with hyperalgesia – R2). R1 and R2 are distinguished by applying additional stimuli on the painful area, either manually or with calibrated instruments to measure thresholds. R1 is explained by convergence of visceral and somatic inputs onto the same sensory neurons (convergence-projection). R2 is due to sensitization of viscero-somatic convergent neurons (convergence-facilitation) and also probably to activation of viscero-somatic/sympathetic reflex arcs.

- Visceral hyperalgesia consists of hypersensitivity of an internal organ, usually because of local inflammation. It should always be suspected when visceral pain is perceived in concomitance with normally nonpainful stimuli (e.g., intestinal transit, urinary bladder distension). It is due to both peripheral (visceral pain receptors) and central (sensory neurons) sensitization.
- Viscero-visceral hyperalgesia consists of an enhancement of the respective pain symptoms (both direct and referred) of two affected internal organs sharing part of their central sensory projection. It should be suspected when visceral symptoms, though typical from one district, are perceived as abnormally intense and/or prolonged in relation to the ascertained disorder from that district. It is probably explained by sensitization of viscero-viscero-somatic convergent neurons.

2.1 Introduction

Pain originating from internal organs may manifest with several different modalities. Careful evaluation of the characteristics of the symptom and of accompanying signs is essential for a correct diagnosis. The main phenomena related to visceral nociception are schematically grouped as follows: (a) true visceral pain; (b) referred pain without hyperalgesia; (c) referred pain with hyperalgesia; (d) visceral hyperalgesia; (e) viscero-visceral hyperalgesia. The following sections will provide a description of these phenomena and the tools for their identification in medical practice as well as a concise outline of their current interpretation (Tables 2.1–2.2, Figure 2.1).

2.2 True visceral pain

2.2.1 Clinical features

This is normally the first phase of a visceral pain attack. It is described as a vague, poorly discriminated sensation: the patient typically uses the whole palm of the hand to indicate the painful area, never the tip of the finger. Its location is along the midline of thorax or abdomen, anteriorly or posteriorly—usually the lowest sternal or epigastic region, sometimes also the interscapular area—independently of the organ affected. For instance, whether the primary affection is in the heart, stomach, oesophagus, gallbladder or pancreas, the painful area is always the same, thus non organ-specific. Patients report a dull, pressing or choking sensation, sometimes not even pain, but just a sense of malaise, discomfort or oppression, which can lead to misdiagnosis In the past, the onset of a myocardial infarction was, in fact, sometimes interpreted as indigestion, especially as nausea and vomiting usually also occurred.

Table 2.1 Classification and characteristics of visceral pain phenomena in the clinical setting

Definition	Clinical features
True visceral pain	Midline, poorly discriminated pain sensation, dull, aching, pressing or choking, with marked neurovegetative signs and emotional reactions. No local tissue hypersensitivity.
Referred pain without hyperalgesia	Pain sensation felt in a somatic area neuromerically connected to the organ, fairly well discriminated, cramplike or pressing, with mild neurovegetative signs. No local tissue hypersensitivity.
Referred pain with hyperalgesia	Pain sensation felt in a somatic area neuromerically connected to the organ, fairly well discriminated, cramplike or pressing, with mild neurovegetative signs. Presence of deep and often also superficial local tissue hypersensitivity.
Visceral hyperalgesia	Pain from an internal organ perceived in association with physiological stimuli for that organ.
Viscero-visceral hyperalgesia	Abnormally intense and/or prolonged visceral pain, both direct and referred, deriving from interaction of two affected viscera with overlapping innervation.

Table 2.2 Pathophysiology of visceral pain phenomena

Definition	Mechanisim
True visceral pain	low density of sensory innervation of viscera; extensive functional divergence of visceral input in the central nervous system
Referred pain without hyperalgesia	Convergence-projection (viscero-viscero-somatic)
Referred pain with hyperalgesia	Convergence-facilitation (sensitization of viscero-somatic neurons) *plus* activation of viscero-somatic/sympathetic reflex arcs
Visceral hyperalgesia	Peripheral sensitization (visceral pain receptors) *plus* central sensitization (sensory neurons)
Viscero-visceral hyperalgesia	Central sensitization of viscero-somatic neurons

11

A typical feature of true visceral pain is, indeed, the constant presence of accompanying neurovegetative signs: besides nausea and vomiting, also pallor, sweating, changes in heart rate and urinary frequency, alvus disturbances. Strong emotional reactions are also consistently observed: anxiety, anguish or a feeling of impending death. This is a marker of visceral pain: superficial somatic pain is, in fact, never associated with any of these signs, while deep somatic pain is only occasionally accompanied by mild neurovegetative signs and never by emotional reactions. In true visceral pain, additional stimuli applied to the painful area, e.g., digital compression, do not normally modify the symptom, i.e., the manoeuver reveals no hypersensitivity. The phase of true visceral pain is not always present in the course of a visceral algogenic process. Sometimes visceral pain occurs directly as referred pain (see sections below). When present, however, it is always of limited duration: minutes-hours, after which it either ceases or becomes referred.

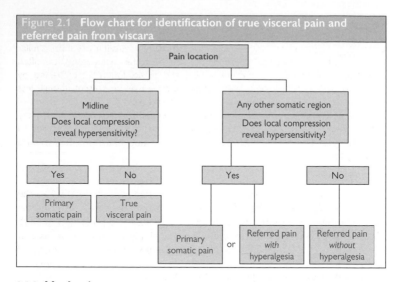

Figure 2.1 Flow chart for identification of true visceral pain and referred pain from viscara

2.2.2 **Mechanisms**

True visceral pain bears these characteristics due to the typical features of sensory innervation of internal organs. The sensation is perceived centrally, as most viscera are supplied with a bilateral or predominantly bilateral sensory innervation (exceptions are the cecum, ascending, descending and sigmoid colon, kidneys and ureters). It is vague and poorly discriminated because the density of innervation of viscera is scarce compared to that of somatic structures and at the same time there is a strong functional divergence of the afferent input from viscera within the central nervous system. In fact, numerically visceral afferents compose 5–15% of the neuronal cell bodies in the dorsal root ganglia at the spinal segments receiving maximal visceral afferent input, but the relative number of spinal neurons that respond to visceral input at this same level is 56–75%. The relative aspecificity of true visceral pain, i.e., the fact that it is perceived in a common site whatever the viscus in question, is also contributed to by the phenomenon of viscero-visceral convergence, that is the convergence of fibers of different organs onto the same neurons in the central nervous system, which has been documented in numerous experimental studies.

2.3 **Referred pain without hyperalgesia**

2.3.1 **Clinical features**

The referral of pain to somatic structures is a typical characteristic of visceral painful processes. After the phase of true visceral pain, or even at the onset in some cases, visceral pain is felt by the patient in areas of the body wall which receive the same sensory innervation as the viscus in question. At this stage the painful areas thus differ according to the viscera involved. Referred pain is sharper, better defined and more localized than true visceral pain, qualitatively more similar to that of direct somatic origin, from which it needs to be distinguished. It is often described as cramp-like, tensive or aching and is no longer accompanied by emotional reactions, but some neurovegetative signs may be present, though less pronounced than those of the phase of true visceral pain. The very first stages of the process of pain referral are normally characterized by the absence of sensory changes in the somatic tissues of the painful area, i.e., additional stimuli applied to the area do not reveal any hypersensitivity and do not modify the spontaneous painful symptoms.

2.3.2 **Mechanisms**

'Referred pain without hyperalgesia' is explained on the basis of the convergence of afferent fibers from viscera and somatic structures onto the same neurons in the central nervous system (convergence-projection theory). The message coming from the internal organ would be interpreted as if it came from the somatic area of referral because of mnemonic traces of previous experiences of somatic pain, much more frequent than those of visceral pain in the course of the life of an individual.

2.4 **Referred pain with hyperalgesia**

2.4.1 **Clinical features**

Later on in the process of pain referral, hypersensitivity of somatic tissues of the painful area starts to develop, giving rise to the phase of 'referred pain with hyperalgesia'. In some circumstances the process of referral starts directly with this form of pain, thus 'referred pain without hyperalgesia' does not occur. 'Referred pain with hyperalgesia' is therefore much more frequent than the corresponding form not accompanied by tissue hypersensitivity .

The hyperalgesia (increased sensitivity to normally painful stimuli), when present, is constantly observed in the skeletal muscle of the body wall area of referral; in cases of particularly prolonged and/or intense processes, it spreads upward to also involve the overlying superficial somatic tissues: the subcutis first, and finally the skin. In fact, it is only in particularly severe cases that skin hypersensitivity occurs, even reaching a frank allodynia (pain perceived for normally nonpainful stimuli), as happens in peritonitic states from painful abdominal conditions (e.g., perforated appendicitis). Vice-versa, in the course of the healing process of the painful visceral condition, the de-sensitization of the somatic area of referral proceeds from the surface downwards: the skin is the first to normalize, then the subcutis, with the muscle keeping some degree of residual hyperalgesia for a very long period of time.

The characteristics and temporal evolution of the referred hyperalgesia have been deducted from a number of studies in patients with various visceral painful conditions, e.g., urinary/biliary colics (from calculosis or dyskinesia);

irritable bowel syndrome (IBS); dysmenorrhea; endometriosis. Most of these studies have employed a combination of both clinical and instrumental procedures to assess the hypersensitivity.

The clinical procedures for hyperalgesia detection are: (a) in skin, dermographic procedure* and Head's technique**; (b) in subcutis, pinch palpation; (c) in muscle, digital pressure. The instrumental procedures involve pain threshold measurement to different kinds of stimuli. For the skin, thermal, mechanical, chemical and electrical stimuli have been employed (via thermal algometer, von Frey's hairs, application of algogenic substances of increasing concentration, electrical stimulator); for the subcutis and the muscle, mechanical, chemical and electrical stimuli have been used (pinch or pressure algometer, injection of algogenic substances of increasing concentration, electrical stimulator). Hyperalgesia is testified by a significant lowering in pain detection threshold.

The global outcome of the studies performed indicates that hyperalgesia only appears in visceral conditions that are painful irrespective of the nature of the visceral trigger (organic or dysfunctional) but is absent in any organic condition which is not algogenic. For instance, no hyperalgesia was detected in patients with asymptomatic gallbladder or urinary calculosis, while hyperalgesia was regularly present in symptomatic biliary dyskinesia. As already mentioned, the hyperalgesia is mostly a muscle phenomenon, involving the overlying subcutis and skin tissues only in more severe cases. Muscle hyperalgesia occurs early in the course of the visceral algogenic process, i.e., a few painful episodes are sufficient for it to manifest, and is accentuated by repetition of the episodes, as the degree of pain threshold lowering becomes progressively more pronounced. Furthermore, it is of long duration: it normally outlasts the spontaneous pain—being detectable in the pain-free interval—and in most cases even the primary insult in the internal organ, though in a milder form. For instance, the majority of patients with urinary colics from calculosis who have passed the stone still present some degree of referred muscle hyperalgesia in the lumbar region months or even years after elimination.

The persistence of referred hyperalgesia in spite of elimination of the primary visceral focus is not apparently observed in every visceral pain condition. An example is acute cholecystitis, where hyperalgesia reverts immediately after cholecystectomy. This finding could indicate that repeated algogenic inputs from the internal organ (as in the case of colics) vs a single acute attack (as in cholecystitis) are necessary to leave persistent hyperalgesic traces at the periphery.

Referred hyperalgesia is usually accompanied by trophic changes of local deep somatic wall tissues, mostly increased thickness of the subcutis and

* For the dermographic procedure, vertical parallel lines, 2cm apart, are traced on the skin surface with the blunt point of a calibrated dermograph at a constant pressure (500g). Red lines appear as a consequence of the manoeuver (vasodilatation reaction), which fade away simultaneously in normal skin areas. An early interruption of these lines occurs in hyperalgesic areas.
** For Head's procedure, concentric lines are scratched over the skin surface towards the area of altered dermographic reactivity, with the tip of a calibrated device, at constant pressure (40g) and angle of inclination (25°). A painful reaction by the patient indicates the reaching of the border of the hyperalgesic area.

decreased thickness/section area of muscle. These can be documented by clinical means, i.e., pinch palpation, but better quantified by ultrasonography. In symptomatic urinary and biliary calculosis, in fact, a significant increase in subcutis thickness and a significant decrease in muscle thickness have been found in the referred area (lumbar region and cystic point area respectively) with respect to the contralateral nonaffected area. Like the hyperalgesia, also trophic changes are set off by the algogenic impulses from the affected organ, since they are not detected in nonpainful organic visceral conditions, for instance, asymptomatic gallbladder calculosis. Unlike the hyperalgesia, however, they are not modulated by the extent of algogenic impulses from the visceral organ. In fact, they have been shown not to increase with the repetition of the painful episodes or decrease with their cessation; they seem a rather on-off phenomenon.

2.4.2 Mechanisms

Referred pain with hyperalgesia has been attributed to phenomena of central sensitization of viscero-somatic convergent neurons. The afferent barrage from the affected organ would change the activity and response properties of these neurons, thus enhancing the central effect of the normal input from the somatic area of pain referral and accounting for the hyperalgesia (convergence-facilitation theory). The visceral input would also activate a number of reflex arcs, whose afferent branch is represented by sensory fibres from the organ and whose efferent branch would be somatic towards the skeletal muscle and sympathetic towards the subcutis and skin of the referred area. Activation of these reflexes would contribute to the secondary hyperalgesia and also account for the local trophic changes.

2.5 Visceral hyperalgesia

2.5.1 Clinical features

This term indicates an increased reactivity to pain of an internal organ, because of excess stimulation or, more frequently, inflammation of the same organ. It is a form of primary hyperalgesia, as it occurs at the site of the primary injury, differently from the above described referred hyperalgesia, termed secondary, which develops in an area other than that of the original injury. Clinically, visceral hyperalgesia should be suspected each time a patient complains of pain for physiological stimuli in any internal organ. Examples are pain in the esophagus or stomach upon ingestion of solid or liquid food when the digestive mucosa is inflamed or urinary pain upon distension of the bladder because of inflammation during cystitis. A typical condition regarded as a paradigmatic example of visceral hyperalgesia is Irritable Bowel Syndrome (IBS). IBS patients experience pain in concomitance with normally non-algogenic stimuli, such as the intestinal transit, or exhibit exaggerated discomfort under endoscopic procedures. Though this syndrome is part of the spectrum of the so-called 'functional gastrointestinal disorders', it has been hypothesized that, at least in a percentage of cases, its triggering event is an intestinal inflammation.

2.5.2 Mechanisms

Inflammation is thus among the major determinants of visceral hyperalgesia. This potent stimulus acts by lowering the threshold of high threshold receptors in viscera, as well as by 'awaking' receptors which are silent in normal, healthy conditions of the internal organs (silent nociceptors). Subsequent to the increased afferent visceral barrage to the central nervous system, phenomena of central sensitization also occur, which further amplify the painful signals and account for the clinical symptoms. N-methyl-D-aspartate (NMDA) receptors have been shown to play an important role in this phenomenon, since NMDA-receptor agonists promote visceral hyperalgesia while NMDA receptor antagonists prevent or inhibit its development.

2.6 Viscero-visceral hyperalgesia

2.6.1 Clinical features

Viscero-visceral hyperalgesia consists of an enhancement of painful symptoms, both direct and referred, due to the interaction between two affected internal organs that have at least partially overlapping sensory projections, e.g., heart and gallbladder (common projections: T5), uterus and colon (T10-L1), uterus and urinary tract (T10-L1).

Patients with ischemic heart disease plus gallbladder calculosis present more angina attacks and referred muscle hyperalgesia in the precordial area than patients with ischemic heart disease due to a comparable degree of coronary obstruction but without gallbladder calculosis. They also report more typical biliary pain and referred muscle hyperalgesia in the right upper abdominal quadrant than patients with gallbladder calculosis (stone of comparable characteristics) without concomitant coronary artery disease. Coronary artery revascularization improves the biliary symptoms, while gallbladder removal improves the typical angina pain. Similarly, women with dysmenorrhea and irritable bowel syndrome complain of more menstrual pain and referred pelvic muscle hyperalgesia than women with dysmenorrhea without IBS. They also report more abdominal pain from intestinal transit and referred abdominal muscle hyperalgesia than women with IBS without dysmenorrhea. Effective hormonal treatment of dysmenorrhea results in improvement of IBS symptoms.

Women with dysmenorrhea and urinary calculosis report more menstrual pain, urinary colics and referred pelvic and lumbar muscle hyperalgesia than women with either dysmenorrhea or urinary calculosis only, over a comparable period of time. Effective hormonal treatment of dysmenorrhea improves the urinary pain, while calculosis treatment via extracorporeal shock wave lithotripsy also relieves the dysmenorrheal.

Thus the concomitance of two algogenic conditions in different internal organs sharing at least part of their central sensory projection causes an enhancement of pain symptoms from both districts. The notable therapeutic implication is that the typical pain from one district can be modulated by treating not only the specific condition of that district but also that of the other organ.

Of importance is that viscero-visceral hyperalgesia also occurs when one of the two visceral disorders is latent with respect to pain. For instance, asymptomatic endometriosis (i.e., discovered by chance at laparoscopy performed for infertility reasons) enhances pain perception from the urinary tract in women with urinary calculosis; over a comparable period of time, they complain of more colics and referred lumbar muscle hyperalgesia than women with urinary calculosis only. Laser treatment of endometriosis improves the urinary pain.

2.6.2 **Mechanisms**

Mechanisms behind viscero-visceral hyperalgesia remain to be fully established. However, since viscero-visceral convergences have been documented in the central nervous system between different internal organs (e.g., afferent fibers from uterus, urinary bladder, vagina and colon converge upon the same sensory neurons), it is plausible that sensitization of these neurons occurs, due to the increased input from one internal organ. As a result, the central effect of the input from the second organ would be enhanced. Since neurons receiving visceral inputs also constantly receive somatic projections, the referred phenomena are also amplified.

17

2.7 **Conclusion**

Visceral pain expressions in the clinical setting are variable. Careful examination of the characteristics of the pain and accompanying symptoms and detection/measurement of sensory changes in the painful area help the clinician in the diagnosis of each specific phenomenon. However, in a large proportion of cases, a single patient presents with multiple phenomena, e.g., he/she may start with true visceral pain, then pass through the phases of referred pain without hyperalgesia first and referred pain with hyperalgesia afterwards. If the affected organ is also inflamed, then visceral hyperalgesia also occurs, and if more than one organ is involved at the same time, viscero-visceral hyperalgesia may take place if these organs have common sensory projections. As a result, the global visceral pain report by a specific patient can be rather complex and its interpretation more difficult. The physician should thus always bear this complexity in mind when facing a clinical situation and systematically consider that what seems the obvious result of one single visceral insult may, instead, be the outcome of several interactions. This is essential for a correct diagnosis and, consequently, an effective therapeutic approach.

Key References

Berkley KJ, Guilbaud G, Benoist JM, Gautron M (1993). Responses of neurons in and near the thalamic ventrobasal complex of the rat to stimulation of uterus, cervix, vagina, colon, and skin. *J Neurophysiol,* **69**: 557–68.

Bielefeldt K, Lamb K, Gebhart GF (2006). Convergence of sensory pathways in the development of somatic and visceral hypersensitivity. *Am J Physiol Gastrointest Liver Physiol.* **291**: 658–65.

Caldarella MP, Giamberardino MA, Sacco F, Affaitati G, Milano A, Lerza R, et al. (2006). Sensitivity disturbances in patients with irritable bowel syndrome and fibromyalgia. *Am J Gastroenterol.* **101**: 2782–9.

Cervero F (2000). Visceral pain—central sensitisation. *Gut.* **47**: 56–7.

Cervero, F, Laird, JM (2004). Understanding the signaling and transmission of visceral nociceptive events. *J Neurobiol.* **61**: 45–54.

DuPont AW, Pasricha PJ (2007). Irritable Bowel Syndrome and Functional Abdominal Pain Syndromes. In: PJ Pasricha, WD Willis and GF Gebhart (eds). Chronic Abdominal and Visceral Pain. Informa Healthcare, New York, London, pp. 341–57.

Foreman RD (2000). Integration of viscerosomatic sensory input at the spinal level. In: EA Mayer, CB Saper (eds). Progress in Brain Research, Vol. 122. Elsevier, Amsterdam, pp. 209–21.

Gebhart GF (2000). Pathobiology of visceral pain: molecular mechanisms and therapeutic implications. IV. Visceral afferent contributions to the pathobiology of visceral pain. *Am J Physiol Gastrointest Liver Physiol.* **278**: 834–8.

Giamberardino MA (2000). Visceral Hyperalgesia. In M Devor, MC Rowbotham and Z Wiesenfeld-Hallin (eds.). Proc 9th World Congress on Pain, Progress in Pain Research and Management. IASP Press, Seattle, pp. 523–43.

Giamberardino MA, Affaitati G, Lerza R, Lapenna D, Costantini R, Vecchiet L (2005). Relationship between pain symptoms and referred sensory and trophic changes in patients with gallbladder pathology. *Pain.* **114**(1–2): 239–49.

Giamberardino MA, Cervero F (2007). The Neural Basis of Referred Visceral Pain. In: PJ Pasricha, WD Willis and GF Gebhart (eds). *Chronic Abdominal and Visceral Pain.* Informa Healthcare, New York, London, pp. 177–92

Giamberardino MA, de Bigontina P, Martegiani C, Vecchiet L (1994). Effects of extracorporeal shock-wave lithotripsy on referred hyperalgesia from renal/ureteral calculosis. *Pain.* **56**: 77–83.

Giamberardino MA, De Laurentis S, Affaitati G, Lerza R, Lapenna D, Vecchiet L (2001). Modulation of pain and hyperalgesia from the urinary tract by algogenic conditions of the reproductive organs in women. *Neurosci Lett.* **304**(1–2): 61–4.

Procacci P, Zoppi M, Maresca M (1986). Clinical approach to visceral sensation. In: F Cervero and JFB Morrison (eds). *Visceral Sensation, Progress in Brain Research.* Elsevier, Amsterdam, pp. 21–8.

Roza C, Laird JMA, Cervero F (1998). Spinal mechanisms underlying persistent pain and referred hyperalgesia in rats with an experimental ureteric stone. *J Neurophysiol.* 1603–12.

Stawowy M, Bluhme C, Arendt-Nielsen L, Drewes AM, Funch-Jensen P (2004). Somato-sensory changes in the referred pain area in patients with acute cholecystitis before and after treatment with laparoscopic or open cholecystectomy. *Scand J Gastroenterol.* **39**(10): 988–93.

Vecchiet L, Giamberardino MA, de Bigontina P (1992). Referred pain from viscera: when the symptom persists despite the extinction of the visceral focus. *Adv Pain Res Ther.* **20**: 101–10.

Vecchiet L, Giamberardino MA, Dragani L, Albe-Fessard D (1989). Pain from renal/ureteral calculosis: evaluation of sensory thresholds in the lumbar area. *Pain.* **36**: 289–95.

Woolf CJ, Salter MW (2000). Neuronal plasticity: increasing the gain in pain. *Science.* **288**: 1765–9.

Chapter 3

Experimental visceral pain

Lars Arendt-Nielsen and Asbjörn Mohr Drewes

Key points

- Experimental visceral pain is a challenge due to difficulties in accessing the organs. However, new techniques have encompassed most of the technical limitations, especially in the gut
- Multimodal paradigms with mechanical, electrical, thermal and chemical stimulations have been developed, being able to mimic many of the pain mechanisms seen in health and disease. Although the methods have more pitfalls than comparable stimulation of e.g., the skin, the more advanced models are controllable with respect to intensity, time, frequency and localization
- Psychophysical scales together with neurophysiological methods and imaging have been developed for assessment of experimental visceral pain
- The current methods are reliable and valid and have been widely used in basic, pharmacological and clinical research
- Viscera-somatic and viscero-visceral mechanisms are important in our understanding of clinical pain and can be evoked in the laboratory together with activation of the autonomic nervous system.

3.1 Experimental human visceral pain research

The ultimate goal of advanced human experimental visceral pain research is to obtain a better understanding of mechanisms involved in visceral pain transduction, transmission and perception under normal and pathophysiological conditions. Hopefully, this can provide a better characterization, prevention and management of acute and chronic visceral pain. Experimental approaches can be applied in the laboratory for basic studies (e.g., central hyperexcitability or pre-clinical screening of drug efficacy) but also in the clinic to characterize patients with sensory dysfunctions and/or pain (e.g., visceral pain). The primary advantages of experimental approaches to assess pain sensitivity under normal and pathological conditions are:

1. Stimulus intensity, duration and modality are controlled and not varying over time.
2. Differentiated responses occur to different stimulus modalities.
3. The physiological and psychophysical responses can be assessed quantitatively and compared over time.
4. Experimental models of pathological conditions (e.g., experimentally esophageal hyperalgesia) can be studied.

As visceral pain is a multi-dimensional perception it is obvious that the reaction to a single standardized stimulus of a given modality can only represent a very limited fraction of the entire pain experience. It is therefore important to combine different stimulation and assessment approaches to gain advanced differentiated information about the visceral pain system under normal and pathophysiological conditions.

The multidimensionality of pain has become widely accepted. For visceral pain the affective component often plays a major role. Not only the complexity but also the subjectiveness of pain perception contributes to the difficulty of pain measurement. This has spawned efforts to establish an 'objective' algesimetry, which does not require the report of subjective states but primarily assesses responses to noxious stimuli in the motor, autonomic, endocrine and central nervous systems.

One further point has often been that the perception of pain cannot validly be examined in a laboratory due to the fact that the pain stimulus used in the experiments is an artificial one. Moreover, the experimental measurements of pain have, as a rule, been developed on healthy individuals. Indeed, the experimental pain stimulus is usually short, harmless, predictable, easily tolerated and hardly stressful from an emotional viewpoint and therefore exhibits marked differences to the clinical pain. Despite these objections, pain has been increasingly analysed in laboratories using experimental measurements with great success in the recent past. This renewed interest has primarily been awakened by the very advanced methodology used in the experimental measurement of pain, which allows for an excellent control of the critical factors influencing pain perception.

3.2 **Assessing visceral pain responses**

In experimental visceral pain studies, the visceral evoked pain reactions can be assessed by psychophysical or electrophysiological methods.

Psychophysical tests require awake and alert patients who fully understand the instructions given and are fully capable of co-operating during testing.

The psychophysical methods are developed on the basis of the psychophysical laws and can be divided into response and stimulus dependent methods. The response dependent methods rely on how the person evaluates the stimulus intensity or unpleasantness on a given scale (VAS/VRS/NRS). The quality of pain can be assessed by the McGill Pain questionnaire which has been used extensively also in visceral pain research.

For visceral pain stimulation it can be quite difficult to quantify the transition from a non-painful to a painful intensity. We have therefore recently developed a visual analog scoring system to take into consideration both the non-painful and painful sensations provoked by increasing stimulation. The sensory intensity can be assessed by a continuous 10 cm electronic, visual analogue scale (VAS) ranging from painful to non-painful sensations. The intensity of the non-painful sensations is scored on the VAS from 1 until 5 (the pain threshold). For painful intensities the scale from 5–10 is used and anchored at 5 = slight pain to 10 = unbearable pain.

In the gut, distension of the stomach can be felt as fullness and satiety, whereas distension of the rectum can be felt as urge to defecate. Hence, we normally use different descriptors for the non-painful sensations in the different compartments of the Gastrointestinal (GI) tract. The most proximal and distal parts of the GI tract have an additional somatic innervation, and this must be considered in the assessment of the evoked response. Hence, in the rectum a combined scale of the sensation of air, defecation and pain to mechanical stimuli has been used, thus relating to the compound functions of the organ.

The lack of specificity, together with the complicated structure of the visceral nervous system, leads to the diffuse localization and non-specific discomfort associated with gut stimuli.

The stimulus-dependent methods are based on adjustment of the stimulus intensity until a pre-defined response, typically a threshold, is reached. The stimulus intensity required to reach the threshold is in physical units, and therefore the use of scales is avoided.

Stimulus-response functions are more informative than a threshold determination, as super-threshold response characteristics can be derived from the data. For threshold determinations, intensity of the stimulus is gradually increased, either continuously or in a stepwise fashion. Thresholds to mechanical, electrical or thermal visceral stimulation are of great value because they are reliably, easily and simply assessed. Thresholds only demonstrate where the pain range starts (pain threshold) and where it ends (pain tolerance thresholds). There is no information about pain perception between these range delimiters as obtained using stimulus-response functions.

Situational and individual factors can influence the pain responses such as diurnal variations (time of day), menstrual cycle, gender, race and ethnicity. Only one study has been published evaluating the variations of all the different assessment parameters following skin, muscle, and visceral stimulation.

Referred somatic pain to visceral stimuli is regarded as a central phenomenon generated by central mechanisms due to visceral nerves terminating in the same area of the spinal cord as somatic afferents. The degree and spread of the referred pain depend on the local gut pain intensity and duration and hence central summation of the visceral stimulation. Measurement of the referred pain area is of major interest as an indirect measurement of the central activity to gut afferent stimulation. The volunteers/

patients are typically asked to draw the referred pain area on the skin during or after the stimulation. Atypical and enlarged referred pain patterns have been found in patients with irritable bowel syndrome, non-ulcer dyspepsia, chronic pancreatitis, grade B oesophagitis, diabetic autonomic neuropathy and dysmenorrhoea. This may contribute to the understanding of the disease pathogenesis in these patients, and evidence for activation of central neurons can indirectly lead to a more logical treatment with drugs directed at the central connections.

3.3 Experimental visceral pain stimuli

Numerous methods to induce pain experimentally are available, and correlations between different methods are often low to moderate, indicating that different information can be gathered. Therefore, it is advisable either to examine pain perception using several pain induction techniques or to explicitly deduce the appropriate pain induction method from the question under investigation.

The most frequently used pain induction methods are derived from the application of mechanical, thermal, electrical or chemical stimuli. For visceral stimulation the adequate stimuli may be similar in modality to somatic stimulation, but the way to deliver them is normally more challenging. Although the adequate stimuli for visceral pain are not fully understood, a variety of natural stimuli are clearly associated with pain from the viscera. Naturally occurring visceral stimuli are hollow organ distention, ischemia, inflammation, spasms and traction. Although we know that thermal stimuli (heat and cold) may provoke pain from the viscera this seems not to occur under normal conditions. Furthermore electrical stimulation, although unnatural, is an easy method to control start and stop of the stimulus.

The ideal experimental stimulus to elicit visceral pain in man should be natural, minimally invasive, reliable in test-retest experiments, and quantifiable. Within the nociceptive range, the response to the stimulus should increase with increasing stimulus intensity, and preferably the pain should mimic the observations in diseased organs by evoking phenomena such as allodynia and hyperalgesia. Some of the existing stimulation methods seem to fulfill these requirements, but most laboratories use their own stimulation paradigms, often without the necessary standardization. The different methods for pain stimulation of the human visceral organs are based on: 1) electrical stimulation, 2) mechanical stimulation, 3) thermal stimulation, and 4) chemical stimulation (Figure 3.1).

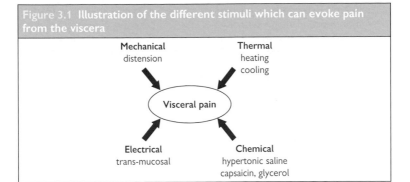

Figure 3.1 Illustration of the different stimuli which can evoke pain from the viscera

Mechanical
distension

Thermal
heating
cooling

Visceral pain

Electrical
trans-mucosal

Chemical
hypertonic saline
capsaicin, glycerol

3.4 **Electrical stimulation**

Depolarization of the nerve afferents directly by electrical current has been widely used for stimulating the gastrointestinal system. The electrical stimulus intensity to evoke pain as well as referred pain is reliable and reproducible.

3.5 **Mechanical stimulation**

Because many hollow organs are easily accessible and distention reproduces a natural stimulus that produces pain in humans, mechanical stimulation is the most widely used technique. Mechanical GI tract stimulation, in particular balloon distension, has been widely used also to study, for example: (1) smooth muscle tone, (2) functional and organic disorders, (3) referred pain and cerebral activation patterns, providing information on abnormalities in central pain processing, and (4) the screening of new analgesics in healthy subjects and in patients with gut disorders.

Early balloon distension studies were based on simple volume and pressure measurements using latex balloons. This caused large errors due to the deformability of latex and lack of control of the stimulation field, and polyurethane or polyethylene bags are now generally recommended. There are, however, still several limitations and sources of error with the systems based on volume and pressure. Most recent studies have used a method of measuring changes in volume of air in a balloon at constant pressure levels named 'the Barostat'. Using the Barostat device, for example, the data must be corrected for compressibility of air. There are four main concerns with these methods:

25

1. Balloon distension in a tube will cause the balloon to elongate to some degree due to the resistance to deformation in radial direction. Volume is therefore not an accurate measure for the distension of the organ.
2. The use of very long balloons is problematic because phasic contractions can be misinterpreted as muscle tone. In addition, relaxation in one end of the balloon and simultaneous contraction in the other end may not be registered as a change in volume at all.
3. Most previous studies have not validated the assumptions on which the data were based. The most obvious and common mistake is to consider the fundus of the stomach to be spherical. From an anatomical and geometric point of view the stomach is not spherical and the wall structure with muscle layers in various directions indicates complex (anisotropic) properties. Distending a balloon in the fundus will deform the balloon into the corpus and antrum, resulting in a highly complex geometry.
4. No previous pressure-volume studies have considered the strain softening effect and therefore it is highly questionable whether the results are reproducible.

Circumferential strain and stress are more likely candidates to elicit pain during distension as the direct receptor stimulus, because the tensile stress and strain in distensible biological tubes are usually largest in the circumferential direction during distension. Considering mechanical and receptor kinematic properties, strain is likely to be a more relevant parameter than stress (and tension).

Figure 3.2 The multi-model probe which can be used for mechanical, electrical, thermal and chemical stimulation of the viscera

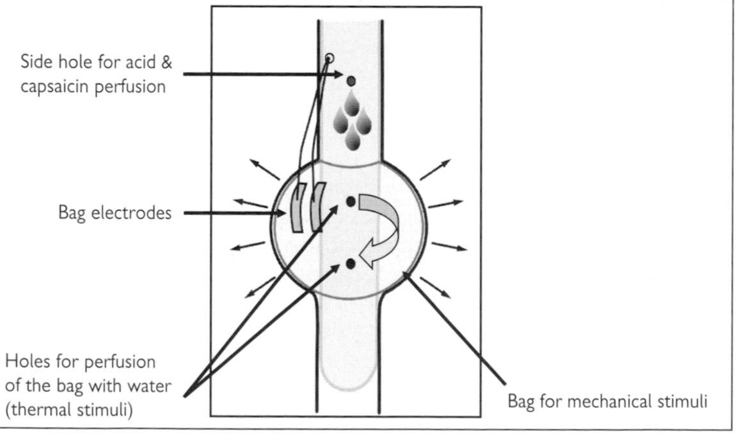

3.6 **Thermal stimulation**

Short lasting thermal stimuli of the human GI tract are believed to activate unmyelinated afferents in the mucosa and Hertz already reported the perception of thermal stimuli in the oesophagus in 1911.

Thermosensitive reactions have been demonstrated in the human esophagus, stomach and rectum. Temperature stimuli in the range that can be felt are normally only relevant for sensation in the upper GI tract and the temperature stimuli showed a nearly linear stimulus-response relationship.

Villanova et al. (1997) observed a uniform perception of thermal stimuli from the stomach down to the jejunum. In previous studies some subjects reported paradoxical sensations to temperature stimuli, e.g., cold was reported as warm.

Previous methods used a balloon perfused with water of different temperatures, but most studies did not perform temperature measurements inside the balloon. In recent studies, the temperature of recirculating water was continuously measured inside a balloon positioned in the oesophagus.

3.7 **Chemical stimulation**

Inflammation of an organ generally leads to altered sensations including pain. This can be investigated experimentally in patients with, e.g., esophagitis.

Chemical stimulation of the GI tract more closely resembles clinical inflammation and is believed to approach the ideal experimental visceral pain stimulus. Most chemical stimuli are assumed to activate predominantly unmyelinated C-fibers (Longhurst, 1995). Chemical stimulation (e.g., acid) has been used as a way to sensitize, for example, the esophagus and hence use it as a surrogate model for clinical symptoms. Acid stimulation of the esophagus is the most used method to sensitize the gut, but chemical stimulation of the gut with alcohol, bradykinin, glycerol, capsaicin and hypertonic saline has also been used in humans.

Drewes et al., (2002, 2003) used a multi-modal probe (cold, warm, electrical, and mechanical) for visceral stimulation of the lower part of the oesophagus before and after sensitization was induced by perfusion with hydrochloric acid of the distal esophagus (Figure 3.2). The sensitization resulted in hyperalgesia to electrical and mechanical stimuli (29 and 35% decrease in pain threshold) and allodynia to cold and warmth stimuli (11% increase in sensory rating). After sensitization, the referred pain area to mechanical stimuli increased by more than 300%, with a change in the localization of the referred pain to all stimuli.

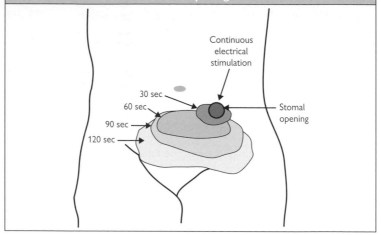

Figure 3.3 An example of expansion of referred pain areas after 30, 60, 90 and 120 sec of continued stimulation delivered to the gut via an electrode inserted into the stomal opening

3.8 **Spatial and temporal summation**

Lewis (1942) found that distention of the gut was most painful when long, continuous segments of the gut were simultaneously distended. Even greater pressures within smaller segments of the gut were not as efficacious in producing painful sensations. Spatial summation is clearly an important contributor to visceral pain mechanisms.

Also integration over time—temporal summation—is important. If electrical stimuli are repeated over time the pain and the area of referred pain increase progressively (Figure 3.3). The same phenomenon is seen following repeated bladder distensions.

3.9 **Drug research**

Experimental approaches can be applied in the laboratory for basic studies (e.g., central hyperexcitability or proof-of-concept studies including screening of drug efficacy), but also in the clinic to characterize patients with sensory dysfunctions and/or pain. In the viscera several attempts have been made to use experimental models in the testing of drugs. Unfortunately, the majority of these studies have used models such as the 'Barostat' in the rectum, where complex anatomy and physiology make the stimulus difficult to control (see above). Furthermore, most previous studies have relied on a single stimulus. An approach to mimic the clinical situation in drug research is to use a multimodal test battery, where different receptor types and mechanisms are activated. The multimodal models have clearly shown their value in somatic pain testing, where single stimuli have been inadequate to test pathophysiological changes and effects of specific drugs. As a further limitation, drugs used in the treatment of visceral pain are often only evaluated in skin pain models. Differences must be expected between the skin and deeper tissues because of the different anatomy, physiology and biochemistry of the pain system in these structures. Therefore, reproducible 'multi-tissue pain models' used for evaluation of existing and new drugs have been developed to combine skin, muscular, and visceral stimuli. In recent studies such models were used to differentiate between the analgesic effects of oxycodone and morphine in healthy volunteers as well as in patients with visceral pain due to chronic pancreatitis, and in our opinion pain models used to test analgesics in the viscera need to be well controlled, reproducible, multidimensional and preferably tested in superficial as well as in deep tissues.

3.10 **Conclusion**

Experimental studies on the human visceral pain system can provide information about mechanisms involved under normal and pathophysiological conditions.

As pain in gastroenterological diseases is prevalent and difficult to treat, pain models may be helpful for developing new and better regimens for diagnosis and treatment of the patients and for screening the action of new analgesic compounds.

Key References

Arendt-Nielsen L, Drewes AM, Hansen JB, Tage-Jensen U (1997). Gut pain reactions in man: an experimental investigation using short and long duration transmucosal electrical stimulation. *Pain.* **69**(3): 255–62.

Arendt-Nielsen L (1997). Induction and assessment of experimental pain from human skin, muscle, and viscera. In: TS Jensen, JA Turner, Z Wiesenfeld-Hallin, (eds). Proceedings of the 8th World Congress of Pain. *Progress in Pain Research and Management.* ISAP Press, Seattle, pp. 393–425.

Brinkert W, Dimcevski G, Arendt-Nielsen L, Drewes AM, Wilder-Smith OH (2007). Dysmenorrhoea is associated with hypersensitivity in the sigmoid colon and rectum. *Pain.* **132**(1): S46–51.

Dimcevski G, Staahl C, Andersen SD, Thorsgaard N, Funch-Jensen P, Arendt-Nielsen L, et al. (2007). Assessment of experimental pain from skin, muscle, and esophagus in patients with chronic pancreatitis. *Pancreas.* **35**(1): 22–9.

Drewes AM, Schipper KP, Dimcevski G, Petersen P, Andersen OK, Gregersen H, et al. (2002). Multimodal assessment of pain in the esophagus: a new experimental model. *Am J Physiol Gastrointest Liver Physiol.* **283**(1): G95–103.

Drewes AM, Helweg-Larsen S, Petersen P, Brennum J, Andreasen A, Poulsen LH, et al. (1993). McGill Pain Questionanaire translated into Danish: experimental and clinical findings. *Clin J Pain.* **9**(2): 80–7.

Drewes AM, Gregersen H, Arendt-Nielsen L (2003). Experimental pain in gastro-enterology: a reappraisal of human studies. *Scand J Gastroenterol.* **38**: 1115–30.

Drewes AM, Reddy H, Pedersen J, Funch-Jensen P, Gregersen H, Arendt-Nielsen L (2006). Multimodal pain stimulations in patients with grade B oesophagitis. *Gut.* **55**(7): 926–32.

Ford MJ, Camilleri M, Zinsmeister AR, Hanson RB (1995). Psychosensory modulation of colonic sensation in the human transverse and sigmoid colon. *Gastroenterology.* **109**: 1772–80.

Frøbert O, Arendt-Nielsen L, Bak P, Andersen OK, Funch-Jensen P, Bagger JP (1994). Electric stimulation of the esophageal mucosa. Perception and brain-evoked potentials. *Scand J Gastroenterol.* **29**(9): 776–81.

Frøkjaer JB, Andersen SD, Ejskjaer N, Funch-Jensen P, Arendt-Nielsen L, Gregersen H, *et al.* (2007). Gut sensations in diabetic autonomic neuropathy. *Pain.* **131**(3): 320–9.

Gregersen H (2002). *Biomechanics of the Gastrointestinal Tract.* London: Springer Verlag.

Hertz AF (1911). The sensibility of the alimentary tract in health and disease. *Lancet.* **1**: 1051–6.

Lewis T (1942). *Pain.* London: MacMillan.

Longhurst JC (1995). Chemosensitive abdominal visceral afferent. In: GF Gebhart (ed). *Visceral Pain.* IASP Press, Seattle, pp. 99–132.

Malcolm A, Phillips SF, Kellow JE, Cousins MJ (2001). Direct clinical evidence for spinal hyperalgesia in a patient with irritable bowel syndrome. *Am J Gastroenterol.* **96**: 2427–31.

Mertz H, Fullerton S, Naliboff B, Mayer EA (1998). Symptoms and visceral perception in severe functional and organic dyspepsia. *Gut.* **42**: 814–22.

Ness TJ, Gebhart GF (1990). Visceral pain: a review of experimental studies. *Pain.* **41**: 167–234.

Price DD and Harkins SW (1992). Psychophysical approaches to pain measurement and assessment. In: DC Turk and R Melzack (eds), *Handbook of Pain Assessment.* Guilford Press, New York, pp. 111–34.

Silverman DH, Munakata JA, Ennes H, Mandelkern MA, Hoh CK, Mayer EA (1997). Regional cerebral activity in normal and pathological perception of visceral pain. *Gastroenterology.* **112**: 64–72.

Staahl C, Reddy H, Andersen SD, Arendt-Nielsen L, Drewes AM (2006). Multi-modal and tissue-differentiated experimental pain assessment: reproducibility of a new concept for assessment of analgesics. *Basic Clin Pharmacol Toxicol.* **98**(2): 201–11.

Staahl C, Dimcevski G, Andersen SD, Thorsgaard N, Christrup LL, Arendt-Nielsen L, *et al.* (2007). Differential Effect of Opioids in Patients with Chronic Pancreatitis. An Experimental Pain Study. *Scand J Gastroenterol.* **42**: 383–90.

Swarbrick ET, Hegarty JE, Bat L, Williams CB, Dawson AM (1980). Site of pain from the irritable bowel. *Lancet.* **2**: 443–6.

Van der Schaar PJ, Lamers CB, Masclee AA (1999). The role of the barostat in human research and clinical practice. *Scand J Gastroenterol Suppl.* **230**: 52–63.

Villanova N, Azpiroz F, Malagelada J-R (1997). Perception and gut reflexes induced by stimulation of gastrointestinal thermoreceptors in humans. *J Physiol.* **502**: 215–22.

Chapter 4

Animal models of visceral pain

Fernando Cervero and Jennifer M.A. Laird

Key points

- Animal models of visceral pain should reproduce the distinct clinical features of visceral pain or approach a clinically relevant mechanism
- Some of the simplest and most widely used animal models of visceral pain are based on the application of stimuli that are not clinically relevant
- Animal models based on the development of primary and/or secondary (or referred) visceral hyperalgesia are more useful for the study of mechanisms relevant to clinical pain conditions, especially those characterized by visceral hypersensitivity
- Several animal models reproduce the features of specific diseases (ureteric calculosis, endometriosis, pancreatitis, functional pain). Disease-based models can help elucidate the mechanisms of the disease that lead to pain.

4.1 Modeling the clinical features of visceral pain

The investigation of pain mechanisms requires the development of suitable animal models. These models should be as simple as possible, fulfill the ethical requirements for the treatment of research animals and reproduce processes and conditions that are clinically relevant. In this chapter we review briefly the various experimental approaches available to study the mechanisms of visceral pain and discuss their relevance to human visceral pain conditions.

Visceral pain has clinical features that make it unique and different from somatic pain. These are: (i) visceral pain is not evoked from all viscera, (ii) it is not linked to visceral injury, (iii) it is referred to other, often remote, locations, (iv) it is diffuse and poorly localized and (v) it is accompanied by exaggerated motor and autonomic reflexes (see Table 4.1).

The mechanisms responsible for these clinical features of visceral pain are also unique (see Table 4.1). Properties (i) and (ii) are due to the functional properties of the peripheral receptors that innervate visceral organs and to the fact that many viscera are innervated by receptors whose activation does not evoke conscious perception and therefore not sensory receptors in a strict sense. Properties (iii), (iv) and (v) are explained by the central organization of visceral nociceptive mechanisms, particularly by the lack of a separate visceral sensory pathway in the spinal cord and brain and to the very low proportion of visceral afferent fibres compared to those of somatic origin.

Ideally, an animal model of visceral pain should take into account these special characteristics and reproduce a process or a condition with clinical features similar to those seen in humans. Some of the most widely used animal models of visceral pain measure simple behavioural responses to an acute painful stimulus applied to internal organs. Despite their popularity, these models may not be the most appropriate or predictive models of clinically relevant conditions. We have termed these 'simple visceral pain models' and describe them below. Other, more sophisticated models, attempt to reproduce a mechanism—peripheral or central—that participates in the processing of painful stimuli from internal organs. These 'mechanism-based models' have proved very useful in dissecting the fundamental features of visceral pain processing. Finally we discuss 'disease-based models' where the aim is to reproduce as closely as possible the pathophysiology of a known visceral pain condition.

4.2 Simple models of visceral pain

4.2.1 The writhing test

This alarmingly named test is the oldest model of 'visceral' pain and one frequently used for screening of visceral sensitivity. It is based on the intra-peritoneal injection of various irritants in conscious rats or mice and the re-cording of their acute behavioural response, abdominal contractions or 'writhes'.

Table 4.1 Sensory characteristics of visceral pain and their related mechanism

Psychophysics	Neurobiology
Not evoked from all viscera	Not all viscera are innervated by "sensory" receptors
Not linked to injury	Functional properties of visceral "sensory" afferents
Referred to body wall	Viscero-somatic convergence in central pain pathways
Diffuse and poorly localised	Few "sensory" visceral afferents. Extensive divergence in the C.N.S.
Intense motor and autonomic reactions	Mainly a warning system, with a substantial capacity for amplification

Table 4.1 is reproduced from *The Lancet*, Volume no. 353, Cervero, F and Laird, MA. Visceral Pain, pp. 2145–48, (1999), with permission from Elsevier.

It is easy to use and a large number of animals can be tested rapidly. These are probably the reasons for its popularity. However, is this really a visceral pain model at all? It is unknown whether the intraperitoneal irritants act on visceral sensory receptors or on other sensors in the peritoneum or other parts of the abdominal cavity innervated by somatic afferents. The relevance of this test to clinical visceral pain conditions is very limited. A variation of the classical writhing test uses hypertonic saline solution, instead of an irritant, to induce short-lived spasms of the gut and a colic type of abdominal pain.

4.2.2 **The Colo-Rectal Distension (CRD) test**

This is another straightforward test with a number of variations. The basis of the test is the induction of a short—typically 30 seconds—and intense—well above physiological levels—distension of the colorectal region of rats or mice by the inflation of a balloon inserted via the anus. In conscious animals behavioural reactions are recorded, in lightly anesthetised animals the endpoint used is motor abdominal responses to the distension and in deeply anesthetised or decerebrated animals neuronal responses to the distension are recorded along the neuraxis. This is a very popular test in behavioural pharmacology studies, allows multiple applications on the same animal and can be easily standardized. Although acute distension of hollow viscera is painful in humans, the relevance of these very intense and short-lived stimuli to clinically relevant conditions is small.

4.2.3 **Other distension tests**

The CRD test is by far the most popular among those based on acute mechanical stimulation of internal organs, but other hollow organs have also been used in similar tests, including the duodenum, stomach, gallbladder, ureter, urinary bladder and uterus. There are variations depending on the organ and the species—most commonly rats and mice—but ultimately all these tests are based on the rapid and intense distension of a hollow internal organ and the recording of the behavioural, physiological or electrophysiological responses of the animal—either conscious or unconscious.

4.3 **Mechanism-based models of visceral pain**

The dynamics of pain sensation include the development of an enhanced sensitivity to pain known as hyperalgesia. Two forms of hyperalgesia have been considered. Primary hyperalgesia occurs at the site of injury and it is the consequence of increased input from nociceptors sensitized by the originating stimulus. On stimulation, these sensitized nociceptors send enhanced afferent discharges to the CNS thus evoking increased pain from the primary hyperalgesic area and contributing to the alterations in central processing that are, in turn, responsible for secondary hyperalgesia.

Secondary hyperalgesia is the result of an alteration in the central processing of impulses from low-threshold mechanoreceptors, such that, these impulses are able to activate nociceptive neurons, thus evoking pain. This alteration is initially triggered and later maintained by the enhanced afferent discharges from the primary hyperalgesic area. Referred visceral hyperalgesia also follows this basic mechanistic model (Figure 4.1). In this case the primary focus is located in an internal organ, where nociceptors are sensitized by the originating stimulus and send enhanced discharges to the CNS that in turn trigger and maintain a secondary hyperalgesic area referred to the surface of the body.

A number of models of visceral pain have been developed to reproduce the mechanisms that trigger both forms of hyperalgesia.

4.3.2 Models of Primary hyperalgesia

These are all based on the generation of an inflammatory state in a given internal organ. A variety of substances have been used to produce the inflammation (turpentine, mustard oil, cyclophosphamide, bacterial products etc) applied either directly to the mucosa of hollow organs or generated in situ by metabolism of a precursor delivered systemically (for instance in the cyclophosphamide model). The objective is to generate an inflammatory state in the organ and test the behavioural reactions of the animal, either spontaneous or induced by subsequent stimulation of the organ. As with most other models the experimental animals are usually rats or mice. The basic premise is that inflammation sensitizes the nociceptors of the organ and generates a primary hyperalgesia state for the duration of the inflammatory process or even beyond it.

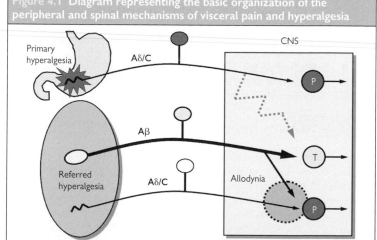

Figure 4.1 Diagram representing the basic organization of the peripheral and spinal mechanisms of visceral pain and hyperalgesia

The diagram shows the afferent input to the spinal cord (A, A and C fibers) and their projection to spinal cord nociceptive (P) and Tactile (T) neurons. Primary hyperalgesia is due to sensitization of peripheral nociceptors and Referred hyperalgesia to central changes induced by the afferent barrage form the sensitized nociceptors.
Figure 4.1 is reproduced in modified form from Cervero, F and Laird, JMA (2004). Referred Visceral Hyperalgesia: from sensations to molecular mechanisms. In *Hyperalgesia: molecular mechanisms and clinical implications*. Eds. K Brune and HO Handwerker. IASP Press, (Seattle), pp. 229–250.

4.3.3 Models of secondary (referred) hyperalgesia

Some models of visceral pain have been developed specifically to reproduce the mechanisms that generate referred hyperalgesia. They are based on the generation of an intense discharge in a group of visceral nociceptors that in turn trigger the central alteration responsible for secondary hyperalgesia (see Figure 4.1). The most convenient way to trigger such discharge is by the application of the TRPV1 receptor ligand capsaicin—the active principle of hot chilli peppers. Intracolonic or intravesical application of capsaicin in rats and mice has been used to generate a referred hyperalgesic state in the abdominal or pelvic regions (Figure 4.2). The hyperalgesia can be assessed behaviourally and lasts for more than 24 hours following a brief application of capsaicin. The essence of these models is to approach the dynamic component of visceral pain that is not necessarily time-locked to the duration of the initiating stimulus. The models offer a long time window that permits substantial pharmacological studies.

4.4 Disease-based models of visceral pain

Disease-based models are extremely valuable to study the specific mechanisms of the underlying visceral disease. Several models have been developed to address painful diseases of internal organs.

4.4.1 Models of Gastrointestinal disease

Animal models have been proposed—mostly in rats and mice—to address conditions such as irritable bowel syndrome, acute and chronic pancreatitis and colitis. One irritable bowel syndrome model is based on the application of repeated distensions to the colon of neonatal rats that then develop visceral

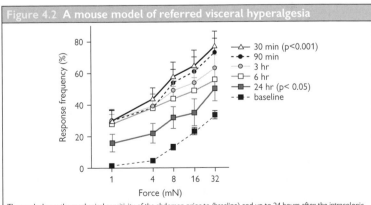

Figure 4.2 A mouse model of referred visceral hyperalgesia

The graph shows the mechanical sensitivity of the abdomen prior to (baseline) and up to 24 hours after the intracolonic instillation of capsaicin. Note the long lasting allodynia and hyperalgesia induced by the visceral noxious stimulus. Figure 4.2 is reproduced from Laird, JMA, Martinez-Caro, L, Garcia-Nicas, E and Cervero, F (2001). A new model of visceral pain and referred hyperalgesia in the mouse. *Pain*. **92**, 335–342, with permission of Elsevier.

hypersensitivity in adult age. Other models of disease of the gastrointestinal tract include the induction of a pancreatitis by infusion of trinitrobenzene sulfonic acid in the pancreas or of colitis by the intracolonic application of inflammatory and infective mediators. In all cases the behavioural responses of the animals to stimulation of the diseased organ or to regions of referred hyperalgesia are measured.

4.4.2 **Models of urogenital disease**

A model of ureteric calculosis in rats has proved to be extremely useful not only to assess ureteric pain but also to study mechanisms of referred hyperalgesia. This model is based on the induction of a ureteric colic in rats by the injection in the ureter of a small amount of dental cement that, after solidifying, is expelled like a kidney stone. The animals show characteristic patterns of pain-like behaviour that persist after the stone has been expelled. They also develop a robust area of referred hyperalgesia similar to the one observed in humans during a renal colic. This is the disease-based model that most closely reproduces a visceral pain condition in humans. Other models include endometriosis in rats caused by the grafting of pieces of uterine mucosa in the peritoneum and models of cystitis induced by partial occlusion of the urethra.

4.4.3 **Models of functional pain**

Functional pain appears in the absence of demonstrable pathology of the viscera or of their associated nerves. It is particularly prevalent in women and preferentially located in the abdominal and pelvic regions. Psychological co-morbidity is frequent and is often associated with anxiety and/or depression. Conditions characterized by functional abdominal pain include Irritable Bowel Syndrome, Interstitial Cystitis and Chronic Pelvic Pain. There are several models based on the premise that major life events, particularly early in life, are important in the etiology of functional pain. Simply applying a period of neonatal stress—for example maternal separation—may be sufficient to generate a state of colonic hypersensitivity that can be detected in adult rodents. Similarly, an intriguing model of interstitial cystitis can be generated by persistent stress in cats.

Functional pain may also be the result of hormonal dysfunction, particularly in levels of circulating estrogens. Models of abdominal functional pain have been developed based on the hormonal dysfunction induced by ovariectomy. Ovariectomized rodents develop chronic abdominal hyperalgesia (see Figure 4.3) that can be prevented or reversed by exogenous administration of estrogens. The hyperalgesic state is characterized by mechanical hyperalgesia and allodynia restricted to the abdominal and pelvic regions and hind limbs but sparing the rest of the body, appears 4 to 5 weeks after ovariectomy and persists thereafter. A particularly prominent feature is visceral hyperalgesia of early onset and long duration. Ovariectomy-induced hyperalgesia mimics clinical observations of abdominal pain states in women where no primary visceral lesion can be found but that show slow onset, hormonal modulation and a trend towards chronification.

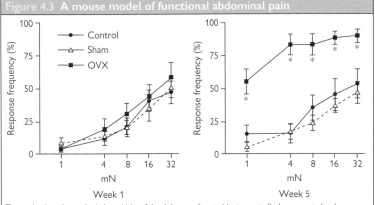

Figure 4.3 **A mouse model of functional abdominal pain**

The graphs show the mechanical sensitivity of the abdomen of control (not operated), sham operated and ovariectomized mice one and five weeks after ovariectomy. Note the robust mechanical allodynia and hyperalgesia that develops 5 weeks after ovariectomy.

Figure 4.3 is reproduced from Sanoja, R and Cervero, F (2005). Estrogen-dependant abdominal hyperalgesia induced by ovariectomy in adult mice: a model of functional abdominal pain *Pain*. **118**: 243–53, with permission of Elsevier.

4.5 **Future directions**

In recent years there has been an emphasis on development of pain models in mice so as to take advantage of the ever-increasing number of mouse strains with targeted mutations that abolish or change the function of specific genes and this will likely continue. This is particularly challenging for visceral pain, given their small size and the relative inaccessibility of viscera. Most visceral pain studies in animals examine relatively simple behavioral or reflex outputs. However, there are a small but growing number of studies employing more sophisticated paradigms so as to access the cognitive and affective aspects of pain sensation, and also to approach the assessment of spontaneous ongoing pain. In any case we should aim to move away from the deceptively simple models of visceral pain based on short lived and clinically irrelevant stimuli and progress towards models that reproduce the dynamic and complex nature of visceral pain and hyperalgesia.

Key references

Al Chaer ED, Kawasaki M, Pasricha PJ (2000). A new model of chronic visceral hypersensitivity in adult rats induced by colon irritation during postnatal development. *Gastroenterology*. **119**(5): 1276–85.

Birder LA, Barrick SR, Roppolo JR, Kanai AJ, De Groat WC, Kiss S, *et al*. (2003). Feline interstitial cystitis results in mechanical hypersensitivity and altered ATP release from bladder urothelium. *Am J Physiol Renal Physiol*. **285**(3): F423–F429.

Boucher M, Meen M, Codron JP, Coudore F, Kemeny JL, Eschalier A (2000). Cyclophosphamide-induced cystitis in freely-moving conscious rats: Behavioral approach to a new model of visceral pain. *Journal of Urology*. **164**(1): 203–8.

Cervero F, Laird JMA (1999). Visceral pain. *Lancet*. **353**: 2145–8.

Giamberardino MA, Berkley KJ, Affaitati G, Lerza R, Centurione L, Lapenna D, *et al.* (2002). Influence of endometriosis on pain behaviors and muscle hyperalgesia induced by a ureteral calculosis in female rats. *Pain*. **95**: 247–57.

Giamberardino MA, Valente R, de Bigontina P, Vecchiet L (1995). Artificial ureteral calculosis in rats: behavioural characterization of visceral pain episodes and their relationship with referred lumbar muscle hyperalgesia. *Pain*. **61**: 459–69.

Laird JMA, Martinez-Caro L, Garcia-Nicas E, Cervero F (2001). A new model of visceral pain and referred hyperalgesia in the mouse. *Pain*. **92**: 335–342.

Lanteri-Minet M, Bon K, De Pommery J, Michiels JF, Menetrey D (1995). Cyclophosphamide cystitis as a model of visceral pain in rats: Model elaboration and spinal structures involved as revealed by the expression of c-Fos and Krox-24 proteins. *Experimental Brain Research*. **105**: 220–32.

Le Bars D, Gozariu M, Caaden SW (2001). Animal models of nociception. *Pharmacol Rev*. **53**: 597–652.

McMahon SB, Abel C (1987). A model for the study of visceral pain states: chronic inflammation of the chronic decerebrate rat urinary bladder by irritant chemicals. *Pain*. **28**: 109–27.

Ness TJ, Gebhart GF (1988). Colorectal distension as a noxious visceral stimulus: physiologic and pharmacologic characterization of pseudaffective reflexes in the rat. *Brain Research*. **450**: 153–69.

Ness TJ, Gebhart GF (1990). Visceral pain: A review of experimental studies. *Pain*. **41**: 167–234.

Olivar T, Laird JM (1999). Cyclophosphamide cystitis in mice: behavioural characterisation and correlation with bladder inflammation. *Eur J Pain*. **3**: 141–9.

Sanoja R, Cervero F (2005). Estrogen-dependent abdominal hyperalgesia induced by ovariectomy in adult mice: a model of functional abdominal pain. *Pain*. **118**: 243–53.

Wesselmann U, Czakanki PP, Affaitati G, Giamberardino MA (1998). Uterine inflammation as a noxious visceral stimulus: behavioral characterization in the rat. *Neurosci Lett*. **246**: 73–6.

Xu GY, Winston JH, Shenoy M, Yin HZ, Pasricha PJ (2006). Enhanced excitability and suppression of A-type K + current of pancreas-specific afferent neurons in a rat model of chronic pancreatitis. *American Journal of Physiology*: Gastrointestinal and Liver Physiology. **291**(3): G424–G431.

Chapter 5

Mechanisms: lessons from translational studies of endometriosis

Karen J. Berkley and Pamela Stratton

Key points

- Endometriosis is a disorder whose signs are growths of endometrial tissue in abnormal locations, and whose symptoms include distressing pelvic visceral and muscle pains
- Surprisingly often, endometriosis co-occurs with other painful conditions in widely disparate bodily regions
- The enigma of endometriosis is that its signs fail to correlate with its visceral and somatic pain symptoms
- Innervation of the ectopic growths and the generation of algogenic agents peripherally likely contribute to the engagement of the CNS in generating individually-different pain symptoms
- Mechanisms of CNS involvement in pain related to endometriosis include central sensitization, remote central sensitization, and central hormonal modulation
- These mechanisms likely apply generally to other visceral and muscle pains, and encourage a deliberate multifactorial approach to assessment and diagnosis, followed by an individualized multifactorial approach to treatment.

5.1 Overview of endometriosis

5.1.1 Signs and symptoms

Endometriosis is an estrogen-dependent disorder that occurs in up to 10% of women of childbearing age. Its signs include the presence of endometrial tissue outside the uterus, most often on pelvic cavity surfaces. Symptoms associated with these signs include subfertility and a variety of pelvic pains. Although both subfertility and pain can occur together, some authors have suggested that the two symptoms indicate separate disorders with distinct etiology. The present chapter focuses on the pains.

5.1.2 **Signs: the pathogenesis of endometriosis**

Of the several theories on the pathogenesis of endometriosis, retrograde menstruation through the fallopian tube into the peritoneal cavity with subsequent attachment of the sloughed endometrial fragments to the peritoneum is the most widely accepted (Box 5.1). This theory is supported by findings that women with endometriosis more frequently have subendometrial myometrial contractions ascending from the cervix to the fundus, have heavier menses, and deposit greater amounts of menstruated endometrial tissue within the peritoneal cavity than healthy controls. The continued growth and survival of the implants occurs in the context of a suboptimal immune response to clear the tissue, higher local levels of estrogens, and involves establishing a blood supply to the implants.

5.1.3 **Pain symptoms**

The most common pain associated with endometriosis is severe dysmenorrhea. Others include dyspareunia (including vaginal hyperalgesia), dyschesia (including rectal hyperalgesia), and chronic pelvic pain. The severity of these pains can, but does not always, vary with the menstrual cycle. Virtually all types of pains are accompanied by muscle or cutaneous hyperalgesia, usually in the lower back, abdomen, rectum, vagina and other parts of the pelvis.

5.1.4 **Co-morbidity**

Another important feature of women with pain and endometriosis is that ~20% have other co-occurring chronic pain conditions, such as irritable bowel syndrome, interstitial cystitis/painful bladder syndrome, vulvodynia, temporo mandibular disorder, migraine, fibromyalgia, kidney stones, and autoimmune disorders such as systemic lupus erythematosus, rheumatoid arthritis, chronic fatigue syndrome, and Sjogren's syndrome. The severity of the visceral and muscle pains and other symptoms of these co-morbid conditions, like those of endometriosis, can, but do not always, vary with the menstrual cycle.

Box 5.1 Theories of the pathogenesis of endometrial implants

- Retrograde menstruation/transplantation
- Coelomic metaplasia
- Altered cellular immunity
- Metastasis
- Genetic factors
- Environmental factors
- Multifactorial mode of inheritance: interactions between genes and environment.

Box 5.1 is adapted, from Panel 1 in Giudice, LC and Kao, LC (2004). Endometriosis. *Lancet*. **364**: 1789–99, with permission of Elsevier.

5.1.5 **Relations of signs of endometriosis to pain symptoms**

Endometriosis is a puzzling disorder because pain symptoms generally fail to correlate with signs. Some women report no or minor symptoms, yet when their pelvic or abdominal cavity is examined for other reasons, extensive endometriosis lesions are obvious. Other women have few or no signs but report extremely distressing and painful conditions. In general, although there are a number of supportable theories concerning the pathogenesis of the ectopic growths, much less is known about how the signs come to be associated with pain symptoms in different individuals.

Numerous clinical studies have unsuccessfully tried to elucidate how different characteristics of the ectopic growths correlate with pain symptoms. Neither the type, location, temporal pattern, nor, importantly, the severity of pain symptoms appears to correlate meaningfully with the amount or location of ectopic growths. Part of the problem has been that the assessment of pain in women lacked consistency and rigor, and the issue of co-morbid conditions was not addressed. However, most authors agree that the depth of infiltration of the implants into peritoneal tissues and the presence of abnormal levels of proinflammatory cytokines, prostaglandins, chemokines and other molecules that the ectopic growths or nearby tissues release into the peritoneal cavity contribute to the existence or severity of pain symptoms.

5.2 **Mechanisms of endometriosis**

Studies of mechanisms of endometriosis are of two main types. The first aims to understand how the ectopic lesions are formed, developed, and maintained. The second aims to understand what aspects of the ectopic growths underlie symptoms. Both types of study are carried out in both women and animal models.

5.2.1 **Studies in women**

Endometriosis has been shown to be heritable with a six-fold increased risk of endometriosis for first-degree relatives of women with severe endometriosis than relatives of unaffected women. The International Endogene Study group has been doing linkage analysis to identify regions of shared polymorphic microsatellite markers in affected siblings. Candidate genes with some biological plausibility have been reported from various studies of affected sibling-pairs and gene linkage studies (Box 5.2).

Endometriotic lesions produce a greater amount of estradiol compared to the endometrium. Implants contain a stimulatory transcription factor that increases aromatase transcription such that androstenedione is converted to estrone. This weak estrogen is then converted to estradiol, the potent estrogen. Higher levels of estradiol persist locally because the enzyme that inactivates this hormone in the eutopic endometrium of healthy women, 17β-hydroxysteroid dehydrogenase 2, is absent from the glandular cells of the lesions. The sustained higher levels of estradiol likely enhance lesion growth and influence the peritoneal milieu.

The peritoneal environment of women with endometriosis differs from women without the disease. In women with endometriosis, the peritoneal fluid has high concentrations of angiogenic factors, cytokines and growth factors, which are derived from several sources. Some are made by the lesions themselves as well as by peritoneal macrophages and other immune cells which are activated in women with endometriosis. Importantly, they also arise from follicular fluid in ovulating women, deposited with mid-cycle rupture of the dominant follicle. Another important contribution is made by endometrium, because it is shed as menses and deposited in the peritoneal cavity with retrograde menstruation.

One hypothesis regarding how endometriosis evokes pain is that it is caused by inflammatory cytokines and other factors produced by the lesions. Thus, some have suggested that the variable appearance of implants and their different

---

Box 5.2 Candidate genes for susceptibility to endometriosis

- Cytochrome P450 1A1
- N-acetyl transferase 2
- Glutathione-S-transferase M1, T1
- Galactose-1-phosphate uridyl transferase
- Oestrogen receptor
- Progesterone receptor
- Androgen receptor
- *PTEN* (phosphatase and tensin homolog a tumour suppressor gene)
- p53
- Peroxisome proliferator-activated receptor γ2 Pro-12-Ala allele
- kRas (Kirsten rat sarcoma 2 viral oncogene homolog)
- Dioxin receptor – aryl hydrocarbon receptor (AHR) and human arylhydrocarbon receptor repressor (AhRR) and aryl hydrocarbon receptor nuclear translocator (ARNT)
- Catchol-o-methyltransferase
- Polymorphisms of genes involved in biosythesis of estrogens; e.g., Cytochrome P450 17 a-hydroxylase/17, 20-lyase (CYP17); CYP19A1
- COMT (Catechol-O-methyl transferase)
- Intracellular adhesion molecule-1
- Interleukin 6 receptor
- Matrix metalloproteinases
- RANTES (Regulated upon Activation, Normal T-cell Expressed, and Secreted)
- Tumour necrosis factor
- Vascular endothelial growth factor
- Nuclear Factor kappa B

Box 5.2 is adapted from Panel 2 in Giudice, LC and Kao, LC (2004). Endometriosis. *The Lancet.* **364**: 1789–99, with permission of Elsevier.

histologic content enable different implants to have different pathophysiologic effects and that altering lesion metabolism may alter pain.

Alternatively, most medical therapies for endometriosis-associated pain function through mechanisms that decrease estrogen levels often also suppressing ovulation and menstruation. As a result, peritoneal cytokines and inflammatory factors produced in abundance during these normal menstrual cycle events are likely created at lower levels. Thus, alterations in levels of cytokines and other factors from normal menstrual cycle events could, in fact, influence central nociceptive systems independent of lesions.

Increased pain occurs in women with higher or fluctuating estrogen levels compared to women with lower, non-fluctuating levels. For example, women who are normally cycling or given postmenopausal hormone therapy experience more pain compared to those taking combined oral contraceptives or after menopause. Neuropathic pain or sensitization of the central nervous system is observed in those with endometriosis, and is suggested by a lack of improvement or rapid return of symptoms after surgical treatment in those with minimal or mild endometriosis. While pain appears to be modulated by estrogens, it is unknown where this modulation occurs (i.e., peripheral tissues, peripheral nerves, sensory ganglia, autonomic ganglia, spinal cord, or brain).

5.2.2 Animal models of endometriosis

A substantive number of non-human primate and rodent models of endometriosis have been developed, most of which have been used to study how the ectopic growths form, develop, and contribute to subfertility. Primate models include species in which the disease either occurs spontaneously or is induced, either by artificially increasing retrograde menstruation, or by inoculating menstrual or endometrial tissue into the peritoneal cavity. Rodent models include rabbits, rats, hamsters, and mice. The ectopic growths are induced in several ways: (i) autotransplantation of small pieces of uterine horn on mesenteric arteries (different species); (ii) autotransplantation by inoculation (different species); (iii) in syngenic mice (no other species), minced uterine horn from donor mice is injected into the peritoneal cavity of ovariectomized and estradiol-supplemented recipient mice; (iv) xenotransplantation via minilaparotomy, subcutaneous injection or intraperitoneal inoculation of human endometrium into the naturally-immuno-incompetent 'nude' mouse.

5.2.3 Relationships between signs and symptoms in animal models

Until recently, none of the animal models presented above was used to study how the growths might contribute to pain symptoms or co-morbidity. Recently, however, one rat model of surgically-induced endometrial cysts (ENDO), in which cysts develop in the upper abdomen, is currently being used to study endometriosis-associated nociception and co-morbidity (Figure 5.1, inset). In this model, the cysts disappear after ovariectomy or natural reproductive senescence, suggesting that they are maintained by estradiol, resembling the relation between estrogens and the growths in women (see section 5.2.2). Rats with ENDO are subfertile, once again mimicking the situation in women.

Figure 5.1 Endometriosis-associated nociception and co-morbidity

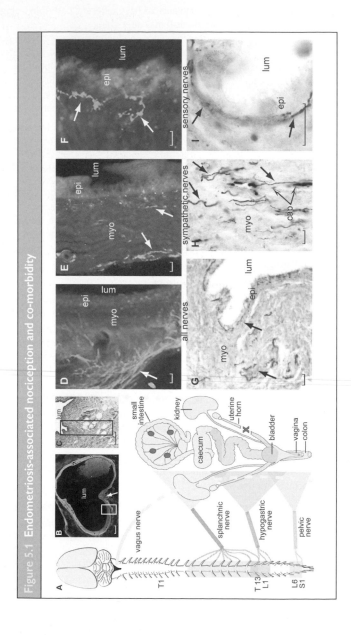

Importantly, the cysts develop their own sensory and sympathetic nerve supply that connects them directly with spinal segments T5-T6 via the splanchnic nerves as well as with the brainstem via the vagus nerve. This new innervation is also found in ectopic growths in women. It is likely that nerve sprouts innervating the ectopic growths are derived from nerve fibers that had originally supplied blood vessels and these vessels branch to vascularize the developing cysts, suggesting that endometriosis may be classifiable as a neurovascular condition.

Regarding nociception, rats with ENDO slowly develop vaginal hyperalgesia over the course of several months in parallel with the growth of the cysts, and the severity of the hyperalgesia varies with estradiol levels during the rat's ovarian cycle. This ENDO-induced vaginal hyperalgesia is also associated with increases in abdominal muscle activity; i.e., referred muscle pain, which also varies with the estrous cycle. Importantly, the severity of these symptoms induced by ENDO does not correlate with the amount of cystic growth.

Regarding co-morbidity, the ENDO condition in rats evokes signs of bladder inflammation and overactive bladder symptoms in an otherwise healthy bladder. In addition, the ENDO condition exacerbates the rat's spontaneous pain behaviors and reduces abdominal muscle pain thresholds associated with passing a ureteral stone. Importantly, the presence of the ureteral stone in the rats with ENDO also induces spontaneous pain behaviors associated with uterine pain, that are not evident in rats with ENDO alone. In other words, pathological conditions associated with one visceral organ can enhance pain symptoms associated with pathological conditions of another organ.

Thus, this model so far reproduces at least some of the pain and pelvic organ symptoms associated with endometriosis in women; e.g, dyspareunia, bladder dysfunction, increased pain from ureteral stones, and abdominal muscle pain, while also reproducing the lack of correlation between the amount of ectopic growth and the pain symptoms.

5.2.4 Potential mechanisms for pains associated with endometriosis

Taken together, the findings discussed above suggest that this rat model has value for improving clinical understanding of endometriosis and pain. Indeed, the findings may already have implications for how endometrial growths might become associated with individually-variant pain symptoms. With reference to Figure 5.1, it is evident that the cysts' location and innervation are remote from the bladder and vaginal canal. Therefore, the most likely way in which the cysts could influence input from or output to these pelvic organs would be via interconnections within the spinal cord and brain, a mechanism that likely also applies to the effects of ENDO on pain associated with passing ureteral calculi.

This situation places the generation of the pain experience(s) squarely within the CNS. The fact that the sensory afferents from the ectopic growths would be activated by inflammatory agents produced by or deposited near the growths further suggests that one major mechanism contributing to the pains is central sensitization, which would, in turn, allow for those pains to become independent of the ectopic growths. Due to wide divergence and convergence of information within the CNS, and the CNS's plasticity and modifiability by hormonal dynamics such as those of estradiol, the effects of such sensitization could not only be remote in time and location from the original nociceptive events (i.e., the ectopic growths), but also variable from individual to individual, depending upon that individual's past history and current environmental and hormonal circumstances.

The many mechanisms discussed in previous sections are summarized in Box 5.3. It is evident from this discussion that no one mechanism alone is likely to explain the wide individual variance in the relationship between endometriosis signs and pain symptoms.

5.3 Clinical Implications

It is evident from discussions in other chapters that most of the mechanisms in Box 5.3 that contribute to the pains of endometriosis likely also contribute generally to chronic visceral pain conditions. Of principal importance from a clinical standpoint are central sensitization, remote central sensitization, and hormonal dynamics, each of which may be triggered by cytokines and growth factors. Individual past history and current circumstances also play a role.

5.3.1 Assessment and diagnosis

Given that processing of information from visceral structures throughout the CNS shows so much convergent overlap, it is clear that when a painful condition associated with a visceral organ becomes chronic, it is quite likely that the individual has pains or abnormal functions in bodily organs different from the current area of prime concern. It is also possible that the originating source of the now chronic problem is somewhere other than that area. In other words, it is valuable to recognize that painful symptoms that a patient reports from one organ may, in fact, be modulated by a condition affecting another organ.

Box 5.3 Mechanisms contributing to the pains associated with endometriosis

- Sensory innervation of ectopic growths
- Sympathetic innervation of ectopic growths
- Abnormal peripheral inflammatory mechanisms associated with the ectopic growths
- Central sensitization in spinal cord and brain
- Remote central sensitization in spinal cord and brain
- Hormonal dynamics acting both peripherally and centrally
- Individual's past history of painful conditions
- Individual's current circumstances.

Thus, during assessment, it is important to take a history which prompts the patient to indicate problems that may seem, at the moment, to be minor for that patient. For example, a woman whose main complaint is bowel-related pain, may in fact have suffered or may currently suffer from dysmenorrhea, and/or headaches, may have a number of muscle aches in abdomen, back, neck, etc. Knowledge of these other conditions, particularly their timing patterns of occurrence (e.g., do they vary with menstrual cycle, or occur together?), can be of enormous value in diagnosis, as well as in strategies for treatment.

5.3.2 **Treatment**

Pain in endometriosis is first treated with over-the-counter analgesics (usually non-steroidal anti-inflammatory drugs, NSAIDS). If ineffective, which is often the case, then hormonal treatments (e.g., progestins, combined oral contraceptives, GnRH agonists) can be added or surgery performed (ablation or excision of the ectopic lesions, sometimes combined with hysterectomy, bilateral salpingo-oophorectomy, laparoscopic uterine nerve ablation, or pre-sacral neurectomy). Surgery may then be followed by hormonal treatments.

Hormonal treatments are effective in most cases for alleviating pain at least over the short-term and possibly long term. Pain usually resumes when therapy stops. Sometimes, hormonal therapy is not suitable for long-term use, and side effects may be intolerable. In addition, surgery appears to be effective at best in 50% of selected patients with deeply infiltrating lesions or extensive disease. Thus, the pains of endometriosis remain difficult to alleviate and better approaches are needed.

Indeed, in support of this conclusion, recent studies by Giamberardino's group have shown that in patients with both coronary heart disease and gallbladder calculosis or in patients with both dysmenorrhea and irritable bowel syndrome (IBS), or in either patients or rats with both dysmenorrhea (endometriosis) and urinary calculosis, treatment designed to suppress sensory input from one visceral domain improved typical symptoms from the other. For example, urinary pain is decreased after hormonal treatment of dysmenorrhea, menstrual pain is decreased after urinary stone elimination following lithotripsy.

This situation strongly supports a multifactorial approach towards treatment that addresses CNS components of the chronic distressing pains of endometriosis or of any chronic pain condition. The strategy is not necessarily multidisciplinary (i.e., involves different types of practitioners or vastly different therapies). Instead it suggests that the pain sufferer be actively engaged in a treatment approach in which pain alleviation is multiply addressed by simultaneous implementation of more than one therapy. Table 5.1 provides a growing list of things, not all of which are necessarily suitable specifically for endometriosis, that individuals in different types of chronic pain can use directly in consultation with their clinician to combine treatments in a manner suitable to each individual.

Table 5.1 A growing list of therapies for chronic pain in the setting of endometriosis*					
Drugs		**Somatic**		**Situational**	
Primary analgesics	Adjuvants	Simple	Invasive	Clinician	Interactive
NSAIDs	Antihistamines	Heat, cold	Ablative surgery	Education	Hypnosis
Paracetamol	Laxatives	Exercise	Excisional surgery	Attitude	Biofeedback
Opioids	Neuroleptics	Massage	Bilateral salpingo-oophorectomy	Clinic arrange-ment	Support groups
Hormonal treatments	Phenothiazines	Vibration	Hysterectomy	**Self**	Advocacy groups
Corticosteroids	**Routes**	Relaxation	Lysis of adhesions	Education	Networking
Sex steroids	Oral	Sleep	Neurectomy	Meditation	Self-help groups
Other agents	Intravenous	**Minimally invasive**	Nerve block	Art, poetry, music, theatre	**Structured settings**
β-adrenergic antagonists	Intramuscular	Physical therapy	Dorsal column stimulation	Diet, herbals	Group therapy
Antidepressants	Intraperitoneal	Botulinum toxin A	Local ganglion blocks	Virtual reality	Family counselling
Anticonvulsants	Buccal, sublingual	Traction	Radiation	Sports, humour	Job counselling
Ca^{++} channel blockers	Intranasal	Manipulation	Brain stimulation	Gardening	Cognitive therapy
Cox 2 inhibitors	Vaginal, rectal	Local anaesthesia	Brain focal ablation	Aroma therapy	Behavioural therapy
$GABA_B$ antagonists	Topical, transdermal	TENS		Religion	Psycho-therapy
Serotonin antagonists	Epidural, intrathecal	Acupuncture		Pets	Multidiscipli nary clinic
Cannabinoids		Ultrasound			

* Table 5.1 is reproduced in modified form from Berkley, KJ (1997). On the dorsal columns: translating basic research hypotheses to the clinic. *Pain.* **70**: 103–7, with permission from The International Association for the Study of Pain® (IASP®).

Key references

Abbott J, Hawe J, Hunter D, Holmes M, Finn P and Garry R (2004). Laparoscopic excision of endometriosis: a randomized, placebo-controlled trial. *Fertil Steril.* **82**: 878–84.

Bajaj P, Madsen H, Arendt-Nielsen L (2003). Endometriosis is associated with central sensitization: a psychophysical controlled study. *J Pain.* **4**: 372–80.

Berkley KJ, Rapkin AJ, Papka RE (2005). The pains of endometriosis. *Science.* **308**: 1587–9.

Berkley KJ (2005). A life of pelvic pain. *Physiol Behav.* **86**: 272–80.

Blackburn-Munro G, Blackburn-Munro R (2003). Pain in the brain: are hormones to blame? *Trends Endocrinol Metab.* **14**: 20–7.

Bulun SE, Yang S, Fang Z, Gurates B, Tamura M, Sebastian S (2002). Estrogen production and metabolism in endometriosis. *Ann N Y Acad Sci.* **955**: 75–85.

Burney RO, Talbi S, Hamilton AE, Vo KC, Nyegaard M, Nezhat CR et al. (2007). Gene expression analysis of endometrium reveals progesterone resistance and candidate susceptibility genes in women with endometriosis. *Endocrinology.* **148**(8): 3814–26.

Cason AM, Samuelsen CL, Berkley KJ (2003). Estrous changes in vaginal nociception in a rat model of endometriosis. *Horm Behav.* **44**: 123–31.

Coull JA, Beggs S, Boudreau D, Boivin D, Tsuda M, Inoue K et al. (2005). BDNF from microglia causes the shift in neuronal anion gradient underlying neuropathic pain. *Nature.* **438**: 1017–21.

Fauconnier A, Chapron C (2005). Endometriosis and pelvic pain: epidemiological evidence of the relationship and implications. *Hum Reprod Update.* **11**: 595–606.

Giamberardino MA, Cervero F (2007). The neural basis of teferred visceral pain. In PJ Pasricha, WD Willis, and GF Gebhart (eds) *Chronic abdominal and visceral pain.* Informa Healthcare, New York, pp.177–192.

Giudice LC, Kao LC (2004). Endometriosis. *Lancet.* **364**: 1789–99.

Kennedy S, Bergqvist A, Chapron C, D'Hooghe T, Dunselman G, Greb R et al. (2005). ESHRE guideline for the diagnosis and treatment of endometriosis. *Hum Reprod.* **20**: 2698–2704.

Osteen KG, Bruner-Tran L, Eisenberg E (2005). Reduced progesterone action during endometrial maturation: a potential risk factor for the development of endometriosis. *Fertil Steril.* **83**: 529–37.

Sharpe-Timms KL (2002). Using rats as a research model for the study of endometriosis. *Ann NY Acad Sci.* **955**: 318–27.

Sinaii N, Cleary SD, Younes N, Ballweg ML, Stratton P (2007). Treatment utilization for endometriosis symptoms: a cross-sectional survey study of lifetime experience. *Fertil Steril.* **87**: 1277–86.

Story L, Kennedy S (2004). Animal studies in endometriosis: a review. *ILAR J.* **45**: 132–8.

Stratton P (2006). The tangled web of reasons for the delay in diagnosis of endometriosis in women with chronic pelvic pain: will the suffering end? *Fertil Steril.* **86**: 1302–4.

Vercellini P, Fedele L, Aimi G, Pietropaolo G, Consonni D, Crosignani PG (2007). Association between endometriosis stage, lesion type, patient characteristics and severity of pelvic pain symptoms: a multivariate analysis of over 1000 patients. *Hum Reprod.* **22**: 266–71.

Vigano P, Somigliana E, Vignali M, Busacca M, Blasio AM (2007). Genetics of endo-metriosis: current status and prospects. *Front Biosci.* **12**: 3247–55.

Chapter 6

Emerging pharmacological therapies

Peter Holzer and Ulrike Holzer-Petsche

> **Key points**
>
> - Visceral pain is difficult to treat and in most cases relies on symptomatic interventions because the causes and targets selective for this type of pain are largely unknown
> - Efficacious management of visceral pain may be achieved by targeting the visceral noxae giving rise to pain, the primary afferent neurons that are often sensitized by inflammatory processes and/or the central pathways and relays involved in the processing of visceral pain
> - Particular efforts have been directed at identifying molecular traits that are specific to nociceptive primary sensory neurons
> - The drug targets on sensory neurons and their transmission relays comprise (i) mechano- and/or chemosensitive receptors and sensors on afferent nerve terminals, (ii) ion channels relevant to sensory neuron excitability and conduction, and (iii) receptors for transmitters relevant to pain signalling
> - These targets will be useful for visceral pain management if drugs can be developed that will normalize the disturbed function of nociception-relevant receptors and ion channels on afferent pathways without interfering with their physiological functions.

6.1 Visceral pain therapy: current and future

The current treatment of visceral pain is unsatisfactory because the causes and targets selective for this type of pain are little known (Table 6.1). Thus, therapeutic advances are badly needed in view of the high prevalence of chronic or recurrent visceral pain syndromes and their socio-economic burden. The availability of visceral analgesics is limited because drug targets selective for visceral pain have been identified only recently (Figure 6.1, Table 6.2). In addition, the utility of nonsteroidal anti-inflammatory drugs and opiates, which are the mainstay in somatic pain management, is restricted by their severe adverse effects on gastrointestinal mucosal homeostasis and motility, respectively.

Table 6.1 Antinocieptive drugs ('co-analgesics') currently in use against visceral pain syndromes

Drug	Molecular site of action	Antinociceptive mechanism
Amitriptyline	Inhibition of 5-HT and noradrenaline reuptake	↑ Descending antinociception in brainstem and spinal cord. Antidepressant action beneficial in chronic pain patients
	Blockade of Na^+-channels	↓ Excitability of nociceptive afferent nerve fibres
Duloxetine, venlafaxine	Inhibition of 5-HT and noradrenaline reuptake	↑ Descending antinociception in brainstem and spinal cord. Antidepressant action beneficial in chronic pain patients
Lidocaine	Blockade of Na^+-channels	↓ Excitability of nociceptive afferent nerve fibres
Mexiletine	Blockade of Na^+-channels	↓ Excitability of nociceptive afferent nerve fibres
Carbamazepine, valproic acid	Use-dependent blockade of Na^+ channels	Inhibit excessive excitability of nociceptive afferent nerve fibres
Gabapentin, pregabalin	Blockade of $\alpha 2\delta 1 Ca^{2+}$ channels	↓ Release of excitatory transmitters
Ziconotide (intrathecal administration only)	Blockade of N-type Ca^{2+} channels	Inhibition of transmitter release from primary afferent nerve endings in dorsal spinal cord
Ketamine, memantine	Non-competitive NMDA receptor antagonists	Suppression of glutamatergic transmission from primary afferents in spinal cord
Capsaicin (topical application of high doses)	Desensitization of TRPV1 channels	Functional blockade of TRPV1-positive population of nociceptive afferents
Octreotide	Somatostatin analogue	Antinociceptive when pain concurs with hormone-secreting tumours; pain due to malignant bowel obstruction; pain associated with IBS; cluster headache
Alosetron	$5-HT_3$ receptor antagonist	Antinociceptive in diarrhoea-predominant IBS in women (restricted indication)
Tegaserod	Partial $5-HT_4$ receptor agonist	Antinociceptive in constipation-predominant IBS in women (suspended in the United States)
Icatibant	Bradykinin B_2 receptor antagonist	Blocks action of bradykinin, the most important mediator of angioedema; active against pain in angioedema

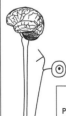

Figure 6.1 Three levels of drug targets on visceral pain pathways and their transmission relays

Receptors in the CNS

Pronociceptive	Antinociceptive
Glutamate-R: NMDA, AMPA, KA, mGluR1, mGluR5	Adrenoceptors: α_2
tachykinin-R: NK_1, NK_2, NK_3	opioid-R: μ, κ, δ
CGRP-R	glutamate-R: mGluR2/3
	cannabinoid-R: CB_1
	adenosine-R: A_1

Impulse conduction and release mechanisms

Pronociceptive	Antinociceptive
$Na_V1.7$, $Na_V1.8$, $Na_V1.9$ channels	$K_V1.4$ channels
N-type voltage-gated Ca^{2+} channels	
$\alpha2\delta1$ Ca^{2+} channels	

Receptors and sensors on afferent nerve terminals

Pronociceptive	Antinociceptive
5-hydroxytryptamine-R: $5-HT_3$, $5-HT_4$	Somatostatin-R: SST_2
adenosine-R: A_1, A_2	opioid-R: μ, κ, δ
ionotropic purinoceptors: $P2X_2$, $P2X_3$, $P2X_{2/3}$	cannabinoid-R: CB_1
bradykinin-R: B_1, B_2	glutamate-R: metabotropic
transient receptor potential ion channels: TRPV1, TRPV4,	(mGluR2/3)
TRPM8, TRPA1	
acid-sensing ion channels: ASIC1, ASIC2, ASIC3, ASIC2b/3	
prostaglandin-R: EP_1, EP_2, EP_3, EP_4, IP	
protease-activated-R: PAR-2	
tachykinin-R: NK_2, NK_3	
cholecystokinin-R: CCK_1	
corticotropin-releasing factor-R: CRF_1	
glutamate-R: ionotropic (NMDA)	
NGF-R: TrkA	
mechanosensitve K+ and Ca^{2+} channels	

CNS, central nervous system; KA, kainate; NGF, nerve growth factor; R, receptors; TrkA, tyrosin kinase A

There are multiple mechanisms that contribute to the initiation and maintenance of visceral pain states. Novel therapies may therefore be targeted (i) at the derangements of visceral organ functions, (ii) the hypersensitivity of afferent neurons, and (iii) the exaggerated processing of afferent information in the brain. Since hypersensitivity of afferent neurons to mechanical and chemical stimuli is associated with a number of visceral pain syndromes, mechanisms whereby hyperexcitability of afferent neurons is initiated and maintained have been in the focus of research. Sustained increases in the sensory gain may be related to changes in the expression of transmitters, receptors and ion channels, changes in the subunit composition and biophysical properties of receptors and ion channels, or changes in the phenotype, structure, connectivity and survival of nociceptive pathways.

Although it is emerging that many relays in the visceral—brain axis are perturbed in visceral pain, sensory neurons stage as the first element at which to aim novel therapies. In addition, drugs that target nociceptive afferent neurons can be configured so as not to enter the brain, hence being free of adverse effects on central functions. Sensory neuron-selective targets can be grouped into (i) receptors and sensors at the peripheral terminals of afferent neurons that are relevant to stimulus transduction, (ii) ion channels that govern the excitability and conduction properties of afferent neurons, and (iii) transmitters and transmitter receptors that mediate ascending and descending transmission in the central pain circuitry (Figure 6.1). The relevance of emerging drug targets needs to be assessed in appropriate experimental models of visceral hyperalgesia with translational validity and in clinical proof-of-concept studies. In view of the many targets with potential relevance to hyperalgesia, the question also arises as to whether modulation of a single target is therapeutically sufficient.

Table 6.2 New compounds against visceral pain currently undergoing clinical trial

Drug	Molecular site of action	Status of development
BIBN 4096BS (olcegepant)	Nonpeptide CGRP receptor antagonist	Phase II (shown to block migraine attacks)
Dexloxiglumide	Cholecystokinin CCK_1 receptor antagonist	Phase II (functional dyspepsia); Phase III (IBS)
Ramosetron	$5-HT_3$ receptor antagonist	Phase II in European Union; phase III completed in Japan
Renzapride	$5-HT_3$ receptor antagonist/ $5-HT_4$ receptor agonist	Phase III
E-3620	$5-HT_3$ receptor antagonist/ $5-HT_4$ receptor agonist	Phase II
DDP225	Noradrenaline reuptake inhibitor and $5-HT_3$ receptor antagonist	Phase II
Melatonin	Melatonin receptors	Phase II (shown to reduce pain in IBS)
AV608	NK_1 receptor antagonist	Phase II
Nepadutant	NK_2 receptor antagonist	Phase III
Saredutant	NK_2 receptor antagonist	Phase II
DNK333	$NK_1 + NK_2$ receptor antagonist	Phase II
Talnetant	NK_3 receptor antagonist	Phase III (shown to be ineffective in IBS)
Solabegron	β_3-Adrenoceptor agonist	Phase II
GW876008	CRF_1 receptor antagonist	Phase II
BMS-562086 (pexacerfont)	CRF_1 receptor antagonist	Phase II
Asimadoline	κ-opioid receptor antagonist	Phase II
Dextofisopam	Benzodiazepine-like	Phase II
SB-705498	TRPV1 channel blocker	Phase II
PD-217014	$\alpha 2\delta$ N-type Ca^{2+} channel modulator	Phase II

6.2 Sensory neuron-specific receptors and sensors

6.2.1 Serotonin (5-hydroxytryptamine) receptors

Most of the 5-hydroxytryptamine (5-HT) present in the body is formed in the gastrointestinal enterochromaffin cells. 5-HT released from these cells is known to target $5\text{-}HT_3$ receptors on vagal afferent neurons to give rise to nausea and vomiting. A single nucleotide polymorphism of the serotonin reuptake transporter is associated with irritable bowel syndrome (IBS), a feature that enhances the availability of 5-HT at 5-HT receptors. Both experimental and clinical studies attest to an implication of $5\text{-}HT_3$ receptors in IBS. However, the utility of the $5\text{-}HT_3$ receptor antagonist alosetron licensed for the treatment of diarrhoea-predominant IBS in female patients is limited by its propensity to cause constipation and increase the risk of ischaemic colitis. The partial $5\text{-}HT_4$ receptor agonist tegaserod is also able to reduce pain in IBS, but marketing of this drug in the United States has been suspended because of a risk of adverse cardiovascular events.

6.2.2 Cholecystokinin CCK1 receptors

Cholecystokinin (CCK) can excite vagal afferents via activation of CCK_1 receptors. Clinical observations attribute CCK a role in functional dyspepsia and IBS, but trials involving CCK_1 receptor antagonists such as dexloxiglumide have not yet proved the therapeutic utility of this concept.

6.2.3 Somatostatin receptors

An implication of somatostatin in abdominal pain has been deduced from the ability of octreotide, a long-acting analogue of somatostatin, to reduce the perception of gastric and rectal distension and to increase discomfort thresholds in IBS patients but not controls. This antinociceptive effect may be peripheral, given that somatostatin SST_2 receptor activation by octreotide inhibits chemo- and mechanosensitive spinal afferents innervating the rat jejunum.

6.2.4 Prostaglandin receptors

Inflammation induces cyclooxygenase-2 to synthesize large quantities of prostaglandins (PGs), such as PGE_2, which are key mediators of inflammatory hyperalgesia. As suppression of PG production by cyclooxygenase inhibitors carries the risk of gastrointestinal mucosal bleeding and damage, blockade of PG receptors on sensory neurons may be a more selective way of preventing the proalgesic action of PGs. PGE_2 excites abdominal afferents via EP_1 receptors and sensitizes them to other algesic mediators. Experiments with spinal ganglion neurons indicate that EP_1, EP_2, EP_{3C} and EP_4 receptors contribute to the PGE_2-induced sensitization of afferent neurons.

6.2.5 Bradykinin receptors

Bradykinin is a proinflammatory and algesic mediator that can act via two types of receptor, B_1 and B_2. While the acute effects of bradykinin are mediated by B_2

receptors, B_1 receptors come into play in chronic inflammatory hyperalgesia. Bradykinin acting via B_2 receptors excites mesenteric afferent nerve fibres and contributes to acute visceral pain, this action of bradykinin being augmented by PGE_2, adenosine and histamine. The potential of B_1 and B_2 bradykinin receptor blockade in reducing gastrointestinal hyperalgesia due to infection or inflammation is borne out by a number of experimental studies. This is also true for the hyperreflexia of the detrusor muscle seen in experimental cystitis in which B_1 and B_2 receptors are upregulated in the urothelium.

6.2.6 Protease-activated receptors

Protease-activated receptors (PARs) of type PAR-2 are expressed by sensory neurons and activated by proteases such as trypsin or tryptase. PAR-2 agonists excite spinal afferents supplying the rat jejunum, evoke behavioural pain responses when administered into the pancreatic duct, sensitize abdominal afferents to capsaicin, and give rise to delayed and prolonged abdominal hyperalgesia. It waits to be proven whether PAR-2 antagonists have potential in the control of visceral hyperalgesia.

6.2.7 Ionotropic purinoceptors

Ionotropic P2X purinoceptors are made of several subunits ($P2X_1$ - $P2X_7$), the subunit composition of the multimeric P2X channels varying in different visceral nerves. ATP released from the urothelium in response to distension activates P2X receptors on pelvic afferents and thereby contributes to the reflex regulation of micturition. Since $P2X_3$ receptors are upregulated in interstitial cystitis and inflammatory bowel disease, it has been proposed that these receptors play a role in visceral nociception.

6.2.8 Transient receptor potential ion channels

Transient receptor potential (TRP) ion channels represent a large family of sensory transducers with a tetrameric structure. Among them, TRPV1, TRPM8 and TRPA1 are expressed by distinct populations of visceral sensory neurons, the 'capsaicin receptor' TRPV1 being the best studied. TRPV1 behaves as a polymodal nociceptor that is excited by noxious heat, vanilloids such as capsaicin and resiniferatoxin, severe acidosis and arachidonic acid-derived lipid mediators. In addition, TRPV1 is thought to be a key molecule in afferent neuron hypersensitivty because its activity is enhanced by many proalgesic pathways via downstream phosphorylation or other signalling pathways. Thus, TRPV1 is sensitized by mild acidosis, 5-HT (via $5-HT_2$ and $5-HT_4$ receptors), PGE_2, bradykinin (via B_2 receptors), PAR-2 activation and nerve growth factor. As a consequence, the temperature threshold for TRPV1 activation (43°C) is lowered to a level permissive for channel gating at normal body temperature.

Capsaicin-induced gating of TRPV1 in the gut and urinary bladder gives rise to pain, whereas genetic deletion of TRPV1 reduces the responsiveness of abdominal afferent neurons to acid and distension and their sensitization by 5-HT and inflammation. Suppression of TRPV1 activity is hence explored as a strategy to treat visceral hyperalgesia, given that TRPV1 is upregulated in oesophagitis, painful inflammatory bowel disease and neurogenic bladder overactivity. One approach has been to dampen the activity of sensory neurons expressing TRPV1 by overstimulation with capsaicin or resiniferatoxin, which induces a prolonged state of 'desensitization'. In this way, hyperalgesic responses to gastric acid and intestinal distension are suppressed in rodents, much as urinary bladder pain, urinary bladder hyperreflexia, pruritus ani and dyspeptic pain are reduced in humans. TRPV1 may also be involved in pain evoked from the parietal pleura.

Since a disadvantage of 'desensitization therapy' with TRPV1 agonists is their initial pungency, efforts have been redirected at developing TRPV1 blockers. As TRPV1-bearing afferent neurons subserve physiological functions such as gastrointestinal mucosal defence and protection from cardiac ischaemia, the challenge is to design therapeutic approaches that block the action of pathologically expressed or activated TRPV1 channels while sparing those TRPV1 channels that mediate physiological processes. This goal may be achieved by uncompetitive TRPV1 blockers that target the agonist-channel complex and by compounds that interrupt the synthesis and intracellular trafficking of newly synthesized TRPV1 while leaving TRPV1 already inserted into the cell membrane intact.

6.2.9 Acid-sensing ion channels

Acid-sensing ion channels (ASICs) are multimers composed of ASIC1, ASIC2 and ASIC3 subunits. These channels are gated by mild acidosis and, as gene knockout studies indicate, can function as mechanoreceptors. ASIC3 may be a sensor of cardiac acidosis leading to ischaemic pain in angina and has been involved in the sensitization of vagal afferent pathways to gastric acid in experimental gastritis.

6.3 Ion channels regulating sensory nerve excitability, conduction and transmission

6.3.1 Sensory neuron-specific Na$^+$ channels

Voltage-gated Na$^+$ channels, composed of a pore-forming α-subunit and auxiliary β-subunits, are crucial for neuronal excitability and propagation of action potentials. Of the many α-subunits, Na$_v$1.7, Na$_v$1.8 and Na$_v$1.9 are preferentially expressed by primary afferent neurons. Experimental gastritis, gastric ulceration and ileitis enhance the excitability of vagal and spinal afferents predominantly via an increase in Na$_v$1.8 currents. Inhibition of Na$_v$1.8 expression by antisense probes prevents the effect of intravesical acetic acid to induce urinary bladder hyperalgesia, and null mutation of the Na$_v$1.8 gene attenuates the behavioural reactions to colonic sensitization by capsaicin or mustard oil and prevents referred hyperalgesia. Nonselective inhibitors of voltage-gated Na$^+$ channels, such as lidocaine, mexiletine and carbamazepine, suppress the central signalling of colonic distension by spinal afferents, and the analgesic effect of the antidepressant amitriptyline may in part be related to use-dependent blockade of voltage-dependent Na$^+$ channels on sensory neurons.

6.3.2 Sensory neuron-specific K$^+$ channels

Pathological hyperexcitability of sensory neurons can result from downregulation of voltage-gated potassium (K$_v$) channels whose function is to repolarize the cell membrane. Some of these channels such as K$_v$1.4 seem to be selectively expressed by afferent neurons. The increase in excitability of spinal and vagal afferents in experimental gastric ulceration and ileitis is in part attributed to a decrease in K$^+$ currents. Conversely, pharmacological enhancement of K$^+$ currents by compound KW-7158 depresses the excitability of pelvic afferents and inhibits inflammation-induced bladder overactivity.

6.3.3 Sensory neuron-specific Ca^{2+} channels

Gabapentin and pregabalin, two anticonvulsant drugs with high affinity for the voltage-gated α2δ1 Ca^{2+} channel subunit in spinal afferents, are able to counteract the colonic hyperalgesia elicited by septic shock and inflammation. The contention that pregabalin-sensitive Ca^{2+} channels play a role in pathological sensitization of gastrointestinal afferents is also supported by clinical studies. High voltage-gated N-type Ca^{2+} channels control transmitter release, and inhibition of these channels by intrathecal administration of ziconotide affords relief from therapy-resistant pain. Ziconotide also suppresses the spinal transmission of nociceptive information from mesenteric afferents.

6.4 Receptors relevant to afferent neuron transmission

6.4.1 Glutamate receptors

Glutamate is the principal transmitter of primary afferent neurons, and glutamatergic transmission in the spinal cord and brainstem is mediated by ionotropic NMDA (N-methyl-D-aspartate), AMPA (alpha-amino-3-hydroxy-5-methyl-4-isoxazolepropionic acid) and kainate receptors as well as group I metabotropic receptors of subtype 1 and 5. Antagonists of NMDA and non-NMDA ionotropic glutamate receptors reduce the spinal input evoked by noxious colorectal distension, counteract the mechanical hyperalgesia induced by repeated colonic distension or colonic inflammation, inhibit the behavioural pain response to bradykinin in experimental pancreatitis, and attenuate the hyperreflexia associated with urinary bladder inflammation. Antagonists of group I metabotropic glutamate receptors (subtype 5) depress the behavioural pain response to intraperitoneal injection of acetic acid.

The utility of NMDA receptor antagonists in pain therapy is limited because of their adverse actions on brain activity. Attempts to develop NMDA receptor antagonists that prevent the pathological activation of NMDA receptors but allow their physiological activation has led to the design of moderate affinity blockers that selectively target the glycine$_B$ or NR2B site of the NMDA receptors. Glutamate receptor antagonists with a peripherally restricted site of action are also explored, given that NMDA and other glutamate receptors are present on visceral afferent nerve fibres. The possibility to control pain in the periphery is borne out by the ability of the NMDA receptor antagonist memantine to inhibit excitation of pelvic afferents by colorectal distension.

6.4.2 Calcitonin gene-related peptide receptors

Almost all spinal afferent neurons supplying the viscera of rodents express calcitonin gene-related peptide (CGRP), which appears to contribute to visceral pain transmission. Thus, the visceromotor pain response to colorectal distension or intraperitoneal injection of acetic acid is attenuated by CGRP receptor blockade. More importantly, the mechanical hyperalgesia in the colon due to experimental inflammation or repeated distension is reversed by the CGRP receptor antagonist $CGRP_{8-37}$. The analgesic potential of CGRP receptor blockade is corroborated by the discovery that the nonpeptide CGRP receptor antagonist BIBN 4096BS (olcegepant) is effective in the treatment of migraine attacks.

6.4.3 Tachykinin receptors

Most spinal afferents supplying the visceral organs of rodents contain the tachykinins substance P and neurokinin A, and tachykinin NK_1, NK_2 and NK_3 receptors are expressed at many levels of the visceral organ – brain axis. While the tachykinin NK_1 receptor antagonist CJ-11,974 (ezlopitant) has been reported to attenuate the emotional response to rectosigmoid distension in IBS patients, subsequent clinical trials of the NK_1 receptor antagonist GW597599 (vestipitant) in a model of human oesophageal hypersensitivity and of the NK_3 receptor antagonist talnetant in IBS failed to show any significant therapeutic effect. Results obtained with NK_2 receptor antagonists or compounds targeting more than one tachykinin receptor in visceral pain syndromes have not yet been disclosed. Preclinical studies indicate that multi-/pan-tachykinin receptor antagonists may be more efficacious than mono-receptor antagonists.

The clinical failures of tachykinin receptor antagonists are in contrast to a large number of experimental studies that attest to a role of tachykinin receptors in visceral hyperalgesia in rodents. Experiments with selective tachykinin receptor antagonists have indicated that all 3 tachykinin receptors play a role in visceral nociception and inflammation-induced hyperalgesia in rodents. These studies have come up with the concept that tachykinin receptor antagonists may target multiple relays in the nociceptive pathways from the periphery to the brain. One site of action may be directly on sensory nerve fibres, given that NK_2 and NK_3 receptor antagonists inhibit the enhanced firing of lumbosacral, but not pelvic, afferent neurons caused by distension of the inflamed colon. A more important site of action of tachykinin receptor antagonists is within the spinal cord where transmission from primary afferents may be compromised. Furthermore, brain-penetrant NK_1 receptor antagonists inhibit nausea and emesis and ameliorate anxiety, depression and stress reactions, which may favourably combine with their antihyperalgesic action.

6.4.4 **Opioid receptors**

Primary sensory neurons express different numbers of μ-, δ- and κ-opioid receptors. κ-Opioid receptors with a peripherally restricted site of action have attracted considerable interest, but their therapeutic potential has not been borne out due to weak efficacy.

6.4.5 α_2-**Adrenoceptors**

Noradrenaline inhibits the transmission of nociceptive signals in the spinal cord via activation of presynaptic α_2-adrenoceptors on sensory nerve terminals. Intrathecal administration of the α_2-adrenoceptor agonists clonidine, fadolmidine or dexmedetomidine depresses the activation of spinal neurons by distension of the normal and inflamed colon. The effect of intrathecal fadolmidine is associated with only minor hypotensive and sedative side effects. This antinociceptive activity seems to be clinically relevant, given that clonidine reduces the sensation and discomfort associated with gastric and colorectal distension. The antinociceptive effect of antidepressant drugs may in part be related to the extracellular accumulation of noradrenaline acting on α_2-adrenoceptors.

6.4.6 **Cannabinoid receptors**

A possible role of endocannabinoids in pain is related to the presence of CB_1 receptors on primary afferent neurons. Activation of CB_1 receptors on the central terminals of spinal afferents inhibits the release of substance P, while CB_1 receptor activation in the periphery interferes with nerve excitation by noxious stimuli. Although activation of CB_1 receptors on vagal afferent pathways counteracts nausea and emesis, a particular aspect of visceral discomfort, the usefulness of cannabinoid receptor agonists in the treatment of visceral hyperalgesia has not yet been firmly established.

6.4.7 **Corticotropin-releasing factor receptor antagonists**

Corticotropin-releasing factor (CRF) is an important mediator of stress and anxiety, traits often observed in patients with IBS. In a high-anxiety rat strain, a CRF_1 receptor antagonist brings the increased responses to colorectal distension down to levels observed in low-anxiety rats and reduces the effect of sensitization by acetic acid in both rat strains. CRF_1 receptor antagonists are currently under clinical investigation for the treatment of functional gastrointestinal disorders.

6.5 **Conclusions**

Experimental efforts to identify molecular traits on visceral pain pathways with a potential for therapeutic exploitation have been remarkably successful (Figure 6.1, Table 6.2). These targets include, among others, TRPV1, ASICs and sensory neuron-selective Na^+ channels. However, the translation of these advances into efficacious and safe drugs has proved difficult. One challenge is to design therapeutic approaches that block the action of pathologically expressed or activated receptors and ion channels while sparing those receptors and ion channels that mediate physiological processes. This goal requires innovative approaches such as uncompetitive antagonists/blockers or compounds that interrupt the synthesis and intracellular trafficking of pathologically upregulated receptors/ion channels.

Key references

Andresen V, Camilleri M (2006). Irritable bowel syndrome: recent and novel therapeutic approaches. *Drugs.* **66**: 1073–88.

Blackshaw LA, Gebhart GF (2002). The pharmacology of gastrointestinal nociceptive pathways. *Curr Opin Pharmacol.* **2**: 642–9.

Beyak MJ, Vanner S (2005). Inflammation-induced hyperexcitability of nociceptive gastrointestinal DRG neurones: the role of voltage-gated ion channels. *Neurogastroenterol Motil.* **17**: 175–86.

Bueno L, de Ponti F, Fried M, Kullak-Ublick GA, Kwiatek MA, Pohl D, et al. (2007). Serotonergic and non-serotonergic targets in the pharmacotherapy of visceral hypersensitivity. *Neurogastroenterol Motil.* **19**: (Suppl. 1): 89–119.

Burnstock G (2006). Purinergic P2 receptors as targets for novel analgesics. *Pharmacol Ther.* **110**: 433–54.

Cervero F, Laird JM (2003). Role of ion channels in mechanisms controlling gastrointestinal pain pathways. *Curr Opin Pharmacol.* **3**: 608–612.

Clouse RE, Mayer EA, Aziz Q, Drossman DA, Dumitrascu DL, Mönnikes H et al. (2006). Functional abdominal pain syndrome. *Gastroenterology.* **130**: 1492–7.

De Ponti F (2004). Pharmacology of serotonin: what a clinician should know. *Gut.* **53**: 1520–35.

Holzer P (2004). Gastrointestinal pain in functional bowel disorders: sensory neurons as novel drug targets. *Expert Opin Ther Targets.* **8**: 107–23.

Holzer P (2007). Treating visceral pain via molecular targets on afferent neurons: current and future. In: PJ Pasricha, WD Willis, GF Gebhart, (eds). *Chronic Abdominal and Visceral Pain.* Informa Healthcare, New York, pp. 245–69.

Kirkup AJ, Brunsden AM, Grundy D (2001). Receptors and transmission in the brain-gut axis: potential for novel therapies. I. Receptors on visceral afferents. *Am J Physiol.* **280**: G787–G794.

Kuiken SD, Tytgat GN, Boeckxstaens GE (2005). Drugs interfering with visceral sensitivity for the treatment of functional gastrointestinal disorders—the clinical evidence. *Aliment Pharmacol Ther.* **21**: 633–651.

Pasricha PJ (2007). Desperately seeking serotonin. A commentary on the withdrawal of tegaserod and the state of drug development for functional and motility disorders. *Gastroenterology.* **132**: 2287–90.

Szallasi A, Cortright DN, Blum CA, Eid SR (2007). The vanilloid receptor TRPV1: 10 years from channel cloning to antagonist proof-of-concept. *Nat Rev Drug Discov.* **6**: 357–72.

Vergnolle N (2004). Modulation of visceral pain and inflammation by protease-activated receptors. *Br J Pharmacol.* **141**: 1264–74.

Wood JN, Boorman JP, Okuse K, Baker MD (2004). Voltage-gated sodium channels and pain pathways. *J Neurobiol.* **61**: 55–71.

Chapter 7

Cardiac vs non-cardiac chest pain

Mats Börjesson

Key points

- Non-cardiac chest pain (NCCP) may be difficult to differentiate from angina pectoris, the most common cardiac pain, due to coronary artery disease (CAD)
- Simultaneous cardiac and non-cardiac causes of chest pain are common
- Always aim to confirm/rule out myocardial ischemia as the cause of a given chest pain episode, also in patients with known coronary artery disease
- The most frequent cause of angina-like NCCP is gastroesophageal reflux disease
- Visceral hypersensitivity is a major contributor to NCCP.

7.1 Chest pain: a clinical challenge

Chest pain is one of the most common causes of seeking acute medical care. Acute chest pain is often regarded as a warning signal for myocardial ischemia. However, chest pain mimicking anginal pain may be non-cardiac.

The difficulties in distinguishing between cardiac and visceral pain of esophageal origin in relation to an acute chest pain episode is clinically well known. In fact, studies of patients admitted to the coronary care unit (CCU) for clinical unstable angina where the subsequent investigation is negative for ischemia-detection ('the heart ruled out') show that a majority of these patients may instead have esophageal dysfunction (gastroesophageal reflux or dysmotility) as the possible cause of chest pain.

It is also known that patients may have two (or more) concomitant diseases/organ dysfunctions, which could all potentially contribute to their chest pain problem. Studies show that up to 50% of patients with coronary artery disease (CAD) also show abnormal gastroesophageal reflux. Also, co-existing cardiac pain (angina pectoris) and NCCP are common.

Therefore, in an individual case it may be very difficult for the clinician to decide which organ dysfunction is the main contributor to the present pain event. This fact makes it important to establish the true cause of a given chest pain episode, even in patients with known coronary artery disease. In clinical unstable angina it is of paramount importance to decide if 'the pain is really cardiac' before any interventions are undertaken. For this purpose different biochemical markers, continuous ST-analysis or stress tests are used, to ensure that the present pain is really associated with signs of cardiac ischemia.

In addition, visceral pain due to organ dysfunction (for example angina pectoris) may be influenced by a dysfunction of another organ (for example reflux disease) via viscero-viscero reflexes, i.e., linked angina. The clinical importance of this entity, however, remains unknown.

7.2 **Cardiac pain**

7.2.1 **Coronary artery disease (CAD)—angina pectoris** (Box 7.1)

Angina pectoris is the clinical presentation of coronary atherosclerosis, a chronic and progressive disease.

Angina is a late and inconsistent symptom of myocardial ischemia (MI), due to an imbalance between oxygen demand and supply, typically the result of physical activity (increased demand) and/or coronary atherosclerosis (decreased supply), respectively. Different theories have tried to explain the cause of cardiac pain in CAD, and possibly a combination of ischemia and secondary chemical/ mechanical stimulation of afferent nerve fibers is needed to reach sufficient activity for pain to be provoked.

Treatment of angina pectoris is focused on reducing myocardial ischemia and thereby relieve pain, either by reducing oxygen demand (bed rest in the acute stage, beta-blocker treatment or regular physical activity to lower the rate-pressure product at a given activity level) and/or to increase the oxygen supply (surgically by coronary bypass operation—CABG and by percutaneous coronary intervention-PCI or medically by nitrates and calcium channel blockers). Lipid lowering therapy, aspirin and low-molecular weight heparins, as well as other anti-thrombotic medications, are used as additional therapy.

Box 7.1 Angina pectoris
• It is typically located as a central chest pain radiating to the left arm and/or jaws and
• Is typically worsened by effort, recent food intake and
• Is often accompanied by autonomic symptoms such as vomiting, nausea, piloerection and/or sweating
• Increased muscle pain sensitivity may be noted in the referred area of pain.

7.2.2 **Refractory angina pectoris** (Box 7.2)

Due to the increasing number of survivors from myocardial infarctions and cardiac surgery, as well as improved cardiac rehabilitation, more patients with established CAD remain symptomatic despite optimal (maximal) medical and surgical treatment. This entity is referred to as refractory angina pectoris.

Box 7.2 **Refractory angina pectoris**
• Clinical severe angina pectoris
• Objective signs of myocardial ischemia on stress testing, i.e., positive exercise test and/or myocardial scintigraphy
• Confirmed coronary artery disease (angiographically proven).

In addition, concomitant diseases, such as renal insufficiency and chronic obstructive lung disease, may also render further surgical interventions impossible in some patients with CAD.

Patients with refractory angina pectoris represent a clinical challenge for the cardiologists as well as for the pain specialists. At present, spinal cord stimulation is recommended as first line treatment by the European Society of Cardiology. Other treatment modalities include transcutaneous electrical nerve stimulation, laser revascularization, temporary sympathectomy, thoracic epidural anesthesia (in the acute setting), gene-therapy, and enhanced external counterpulsation.

7.2.3 **Syndrome X** (Box 7.3)

Box 7.3 **Syndrome X**
• The presence of clinical anginal pain
• A positive cardiac stress test indicating ischemia and
• A normal coronary angiogram.

The majority of patients with syndrome X are women. The pathogenesis is most probably heterogenous, with subjects ranging from individuals with myocardial ischemia of smaller vessels (microvascular angina) to NCCP-patients with a false positive exercise test. A subset of these patients show visceral cardiac hypersensitivity ('sensitive heart'), which may also involve other organs.

Chest pain in patients with a normal coronary angiography is associated with higher scores for somatization, anxiety and panic-disorder. The prognosis of syndrome X is excellent regarding mortality but poor regarding pain relief and quality of life. Treatment options have traditionally been limited to symptomatic pharmacological interventions with nitrates and calcium-channel blockers. However, the emerging knowledge of the heterogenous nature of this entity paves the way for new treatment modalities including treatment of esophageal dysfunction (if present), spinal cord stimulation, behavioral treatment and increased physical activity.

7.3 Non cardiac chest pain—NCCP

NCCP is usually defined as long-lasting angina-like chest pain without any (known) cardiac abnormality. Clinically, it is important to thoroughly exclude a cardiac origin of pain as well as to identify the possible non-cardiac cause of pain.

7.3.1 Gastroesophageal reflux disease (GORD)

Is the most common cause of angina-like chest pain in the clinical setting and is characterized by an excessive amount of acid refluxed into the oesophagus. 24-hour pH measurements are the diagnostic standard in chest pain patients (>4% of recorded time with pH<4.0). Endoscopic esophagitis confirms the diagnosis, although a negative endoscopy does not rule out GORD.

Symptoms of GORD include acid regurgitation ('heart burn'), dyspepsia and chest discomfort. In fact, up to 10% of reflux patients have chest pain as the only presenting symptom, but many also have 'silent reflux'. Patients with non-erosive gastroesophageal reflux disease (NERD) frequently experience atypical reflux symptoms, including chest pain.

In a study of patients admitted to the coronary care unit with suspected unstable angina pectoris, 50% of patients without signs of cardiac ischemia, were found to have GORD. Acid suppression by proton pump inhibitors (PPI) is first-line treatment. Other treatments include weight loss and lifting the top-end of the bed slightly to reduce reflux.

7.3.2 Esophageal dysmotility (motor disturbances)

The esophageal manometric curve obtained during swallowing identifies several dysmotilities, including hypertensive lower esophageal sphincter, diffuse esophageal spasm and nutcracker oesophagus. All of these entities are associated with chest pain, although the causality remains to be elucidated.

Nutcracker oesophagus (NE), the dysmotility most commonly associated with chest pain, is found in 10-15% of patients referred because of chest pain. NE is characterized by high amplitude (>180 mmHg) esophageal peristalsis with a normal propagation. Dysphagia and chest pain are the chief complaints in NE.

While the pathophysiology is unknown, an association between NE and reflux has been proposed, but the first randomized placebo-controlled cross-over study on PPI treatment failed to show a clinical effect on pain. However, it remains clinically important to treat any co-existing GORD. Nitrates and calcium-channel blockers are often tried; these may reduce the amplitude of the peristaltic waves but show mixed efficacy on pain.

7.3.3 Irritable oesophagus

Using different provocation methods, a subset of patients with chest pain of unknown origin can be identified as having an increased esophageal sensitivity for acid-provocation, mechanical balloon distention and/or both. They are frequently referred to as having 'irritable oesophagus'.

These patients constitute a subset of patients with NCCP with visceral hypersensitivity and show clinical similarities, or even overlapping, with the patients defined above as having syndrome X. Clinically it is important to remember that visceral hypersensitivity in a given patient may also involve other organs, which has been shown in patients with irritable colon, dyspepsia and the 'sensitive heart'.

7.3.4 **Chest pain from other viscera**

The chest pain of *lung diseases* may be accompanied by associated symptoms, such as fever or dyspnea, or be related to breathing (i.e., pneumonia, pleuritis).

Dysfunctions of abdominal viscera, i.e., gastritis, gallstones, cholecystitis, pancreatitis and even colon pain, may present clinically as chest pain, partly due to referral of pain.

7.4 **Cardiac vs non-cardiac chest pain**

7.4.1 **Cardiac OR non-cardiac chest pain**

Anginal pain and esophageal pain may be almost impossible to differentiate clinically. They may show similar referral patterns and are accompanied by similar motor reflex activity. In other cases of visceral chest pain, for instance involving the lungs, differentiation may be easier.

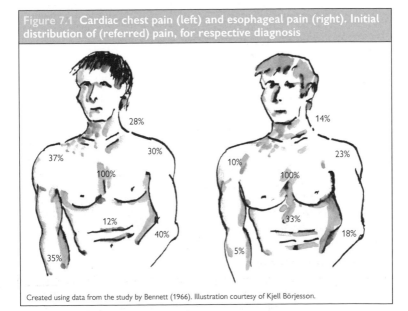

Figure 7.1 Cardiac chest pain (left) and esophageal pain (right). Initial distribution of (referred) pain, for respective diagnosis

Created using data from the study by Bennett (1966). Illustration courtesy of Kjell Börjesson.

Pain is of limited importance as a warning signal of myocardial ischemia. Clinically additional on-line ischemia detection (by vectorcardiography or similar ST-analysis) and biochemical markers (troponins and CK-MB indicating myocardial cell damage) are routinely needed. To increase the diagnostic yield, myocardial oxygen demand may be increased by provocative testing with exercise test, stress-echocardiography and/or myocardial scintigraphy. Angina pectoris is a clinical diagnosis, but it is important to always confirm/rule out the presence of myocardial ischemia.

7.4.2 **Cardiac AND non-cardiac pain**

Many patients suffer from simultaneous dysfunctions of two viscera (for example cardiac and esophageal), making it even harder to distinguish the real/main source of pain.

About half of the patients with CAD may also suffer from GORD. Treatment of angina with nitrates and beta-blockers may increase any co-existing reflux by lowering the lower esophageal sphincter (LES) pressure. In addition, reflux may lower the anginal threshold on exercise-test.

Figure 7.2 Schematic illustration of possible viscero-visceral reflexes between the heart and the oesophagus at different levels

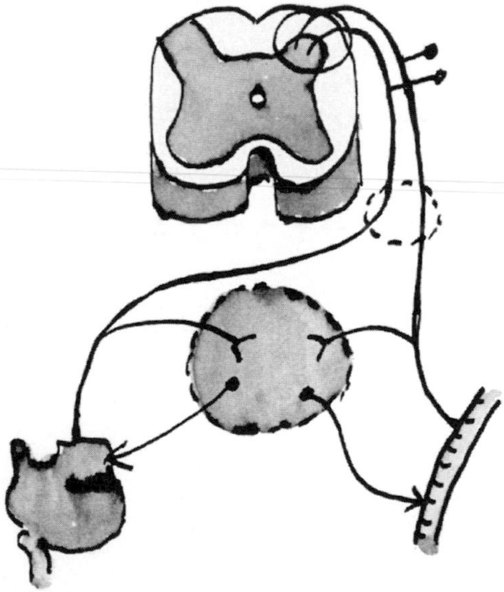

Illustration is reproduced courtesy of Kjell Borjesson.

7.4.3 **Linked angina**

Viscero-visceral reflexes have been shown to exist between several organs. Acid instillation in the distal oesophagus gave rise to constriction of the coronary arteries in dogs and decreased coronary blood flow velocity in humans, confirming the presence of an esophago-cardiac reflex, i.e., linked angina.

The clinical importance of this phenomenon remains unknown. However, in a recent study, acid suppressive treatment in patients with GORD and CAD improved the exercise test within two weeks, supporting the concept of linked angina.

Clinically it is important to always confirm/rule out the presence of myocardial ischemia in patients referred for chest pain of presumed cardiac origin, even in the presence of known CAD. This is especially important before any (new) cardiac intervention is undertaken. In patients with several earlier visits for presumed cardiac pain without evidence of ischemia, other alternative non-cardiac sources of chest pain must be considered.

Key references

Bennett JR, Atkinson M (1966). The differentiation between oesophageal and cardiac pain. *Lancet.* **2**: 1123–27.

Börjesson M, Pilhall M, Eliasson T, Dellborg M, Rolny P, Mannheimer C (1998). Esophageal dysfunction in syndrome X. *Am J Cardiol.* **82**: 1187–91.

Börjesson M, Dellborg M (2003). Before intervention-is the pain really cardiac? *Sc Cardiovasc J.* **37**: 124–7.

Cannon RO (1995). The sensitive heart. A syndrome of abnormal cardiac pain perception. *JAMA.* **273**(11): 883–7.

Chauhan A, Petch MC, Schofield PM (1993). Effect of oesophageal acid instillation on coronary blood flow. *Lancet.* **341**: 1309–10.

Dellborg M, Malmberg K, Rydén L, Svensson A-M, Swedberg K (1995). Dynamic on-line vectorcardiography improves and simplifies in hospital ischemia monitoring of patients with unstable angina. *J A C C.* **26**: 1501–7.

Gowda RM, Khan IA, Punukollu G, Vasavada BC, Nair CK (2005). Treatment of refractory angina pectoris. *Int J Cardiol.* **101**: 1–7.

Hewson EG, Dalton CB, Hackshaw BT, Wu WC, Richter JE (1990). The prevalence of abnormal esophageal test results in patients with cardiovascular disease and unexplained chest pain. *Arch Intern Med.* **150**: 965–9.

Malliani A (1995). The conceptualization of cardiac pain as a nonspecific and unreliable alarm system. In: GF Gebhart (ed). *Visceral Pain.* IASP Press, Seattle, pp. 63–74.

Mannheimer C, Eliasson T, Augustinsson LE, Blomstrand C, Emanuelsson H, Larsson S, et al. (1998). Electrical stimulation versus coronary artery bypass surgery in severe angina pectoris: the ESBY study. *Circulation.* **97**: 1157–63.

Mannheimer C, Camici P, Chester MR, Collins A, DeJongste M, Eliasson T *et al.* (2002). The problem of chronic refractory angina: report from the ESC Joint Study Group on the treatment of rafractory angina. *Eur Heart J.* **23**: 355–70.

Maseri A, Crea F, Kaski JC, Davies G (1992). Mechanisms and significance of cardiac ischemic pain. *Prog Cardiovasc Dis.* **35**(1): 1–18.

Quigley EM (2005). The spectrum of GORD: a new perspective. *Drugs Today.* **41**: suppl B:3–6.

Reyes E, Underwood SR (2006). Myocardial perfusion scintigraphy: an important step between clinical assessment and coronary angiography in patients with stable chest pain. *Eur Heart J.* **27**: 3–4.

Schultz T, Mannheimer C, Dellborg M, Pilhall M, Börjesson M (2008). High prevalence of gastroesophageal reflux in patients with clinical unstable angina and known coronary artery disease. *Acute Cardiac Care.* **10**(1): 37–42.

Trimble KC, Pryde A, Heading RC (1995). Lowered oesophageal sensory thresholds in patients with symptomatic but not excess gastro-oesophageal reflux: evidence for a spectrum of visceral sensitivity in GORD. *Gut.* **37**: 7–12.

Chapter 8

Gastrointestinal pain

Lukas Van Oudenhove and Qasim Aziz

Key points

- Gastrointestinal pain is a key symptom of Functional Gastrointestinal Disorders (FGID) including Irritable Bowel Syndrome (IBS) and Functional Dyspepsia (FD)
- Gastrointestinal pain is a biopsychosocial phenomenon and the bidirectional neural pathways between the gastrointestinal tract and the brain ('brain-gut axis') provide a biological substrate that allows integration of these multiple dimensions
- Gastrointestinal pain may result from increased afferent signalling arising at the level of the gut, abnormal processing of (normal) afferent signals at the level of the central nervous system (spinal cord and brain), or abnormal activation of descending modulatory pathways, or a combination of these mechanisms
- There is increasing evidence that psychological factors (affective as well as cognitive) can modulate brain processing of gastrointestinal signals as well as influence descending pain modulation, providing a neurobiological substrate for a role of psychosocial factors in FGID
- Treatment of gastrointestinal pain as a symptom of FGID should therefore be biopsychosocial in nature, with anti-hyperalgesic drugs including antidepressants and psychotherapy being some of the treatment options.

Functional Gastrointestinal Disorders (FGID), with gastrointestinal pain being one of the core symptoms, are a prevalent and challenging phenomenon for both general and specialist clinicians. Recent evidence, including functional brain imaging studies of the 'brain-gut axis' (BGA), confirms the biopsychosocial nature of gastrointestinal pain and provides a rationale for multidisciplinary treatment of these complex disorders.

8.1 **Introduction**

8.1.1 **Gastrointestinal pain as a core symptom of FGID**

FGID are defined as the presence of abdominal symptoms that cannot be sufficiently explained by 'structural disease'. The symptoms are believed to be caused by a 'functional disturbance' of the gastrointestinal tract, including abnormal sensitivity or motility. The pathophysiology of FGID is likely to be heterogeneous. Irritable bowel syndrome (IBS) and functional dyspepsia (FD) are the most prevalent FGID, with prevalences of up to 40% in the general population. The recently revised diagnostic criteria ('Rome III') define Functional Abdominal Pain Syndrome as a less common separate entity within the FGID: symptoms are largely unrelated to food intake and defecation, and comorbidity with psychiatric disorders is higher.

8.1.2 **The role of psychosocial factors and psychiatric comorbidity in FGID**

Comorbidity of FGID with psychiatric disorders is high, as well as the prevalence of psychosocial abnormalities including a history of abuse. Whether these psychosocial factors play a central role in the onset, course and treatment response of FGID or only drive health-care seeking remains a matter of debate. However, evidence for a direct influence of psychological factors on gastro-intestinal sensorimotor function and symptom perception in FGID is growing. The BGA (bidirectional pathways linking the brain and the gastrointestinal tract) allows us to understand this putative role of psychological factors, which may exert their effect at several levels of the BGA (Figure 8.1).

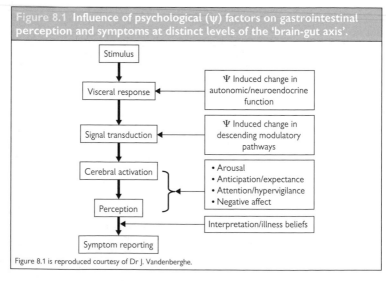

Figure 8.1 Influence of psychological (ψ) factors on gastrointestinal perception and symptoms at distinct levels of the 'brain-gut axis'.

Figure 8.1 is reproduced courtesy of Dr J. Vandenberghe.

8.2 The brain-gut axis in health

8.2.1 Afferent pathways

8.2.1.1 *Vagal afferents (Figure 8.2)*

Vagal afferents mainly transmit sensory signals within the non-painful physiological range. Primary afferents run in the vagus nerve, projecting to the nucleus of the solitary tract (NTS). Secondary afferents project from the NTS to the thalamus (some via the parabrachial nucleus) as well as to the hypothalamus, locus coeruleus (LC)-amygdala system and periaqueductal grey (PAG). These subcortical brain regions are known as the Emotional Motor System (EMS) and play a role in arousal, autonomic, neuroendocrine, emotional and behavioural responses to visceral sensory information. From the thalamus, third order afferents relay gastrointestinal sensory information to the cortical 'visceral sensory neuromatrix'.

8.2.1.2 *Spinal afferents (Figures 8.2 and 8.3a)*

Spinal afferents mainly transmit painful visceral sensory signals. Primary spinal afferents project to the dorsal horn of the spinal cord. Secondary neurons project to the brain through the spinal cord in several distinct pathways. The spinoreticular, spinomesencephalic and spinohypothalamic tracts are mainly involved in reflexive/unconscious/automatic responses to GI sensory input (arousal, autonomic responses, prototype emotional and behavioural responses). The spinothalamic tract projects to the sensory thalamus, from which tertiary neurons relay GI sensory signals to cortical 'visceral sensory neuromatrix'.

8.2.2 The cortical 'visceral sensory neuromatrix' (Figures 8.2 and 8.3a)

The primary and secondary somatosensory cortices (SI/SII) ('lateral pain system') encode intensity and localisation of (visceral) stimuli (sensory-discriminative pain dimension).

The anterior and mid-cingulate cortex (ACC/MCC) ('medial pain system'), with its different subregions, is involved in the affective-motivational ('pain unpleasantness', pain-related anxiety) and cognitive-evaluative (anticipation, attention) dimensions of visceral pain. This complex region also generates autonomic, emotional, behavioural and descending modulatory responses.

The insula ('interoceptive cortex') integrates multimodal sensory and emotional information, thereby representing the internal state of the organism. It sends efferent projections to the EMS, providing a substrate of higher-order control of autonomic visceromotor responses.

The prefrontal cortex (PFC), with its different subdivisions, mainly plays a role in cognitive influences on pain, (secondary) pain affect and endogenous antinociceptive responses. It is also involved in selecting and generating responses to visceral sensory input.

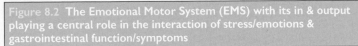

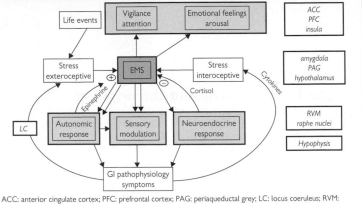

ACC: anterior cingulate cortex; PFC: prefrontal cortex; PAG: periaqueductal grey; LC: locus coeruleus; RVM: rostrolateral ventral medulla.
Figure 8.2 is adapted with permission from Meyer EA, Gut. (2000).

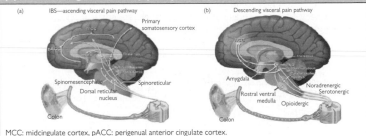

MCC: midcingulate cortex, pACC: perigenual anterior cingulate cortex.
ACC: anterior cingulate cortex, PAG: periaqueductal grey.
Figure 8.3 is reproduced with permission from Drossman DA, *Clin Gastroenterol Hepatol*. (2004).

8.2.3 **Descending modulation (Figure 8.3b)**

The ACC is the central cortical region involved in descending modulatory control of GI pain, with its efferent output to the EMS in general and the PAG in particular. Thus, the ACC may be the neurobiological substrate of cognitive and affective influences on pain transmission. The EMS structures send descending projections to the monoaminergic brainstem nuclei [locus coeruleus (noradrenaline), raphe nuclei (serotonin) and rostrolateral ventral medulla], which in turn send descending output to the dorsal horn of the spinal cord, influencing the synaptic transmission of GI sensory signals at this level ('gate mechanism'). Endogenous opioids are crucially involved in descending modulation at all levels, together with the monamines mentioned above.

8.2.4 **Psychological modulation of visceral sensory information processing**

Functional brain imaging studies in healthy volunteers have shown that affective (emotional context created by fearful facial expressions) and cognitive factors (including selective or divided attention, anticipation and classical conditioning phenomena) are able to modulate brain processing of GI distension as well as the intensity of the symptoms arising from it. This modulation mainly occurs at the level of the ACC, insula and prefrontal cortex.

8.3 **The brain-gut axis and the origin of gastrointestinal pain in FGID**

Gastrointestinal pain in FGID may theoretically be caused by heightened afferent input arising at the level of the gut, abnormal central nervous system (both spinal cord and brain) processing of (normal) visceral afferent input (which may be caused by psychological factors, see above) and/or aberrant

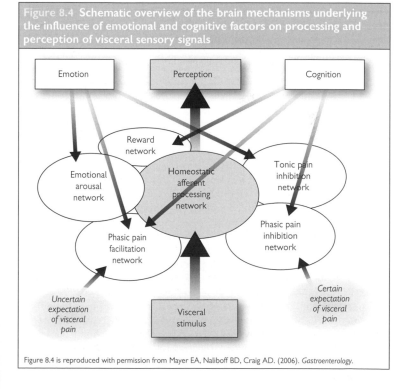

Figure 8.4 Schematic overview of the brain mechanisms underlying the influence of emotional and cognitive factors on processing and perception of visceral sensory signals

Figure 8.4 is reproduced with permission from Mayer EA, Naliboff BD, Craig AD. (2006). *Gastroenterology.*

75

descending modulatory responses to visceral sensory information (which may also be under psychological influence) (Figure 8.4). Given the heterogeneous nature of FGID, it is likely that a complex combination of these mechanisms gives rise to gastrointestinal pain, although the relative contribution of each mechanism may vary between patients.

8.3.1 **Gastrointestinal sensorimotor dysfunction in FGID**

FGID patients as a group show abnormalities in GI motor (colonic motility in IBS, gastric accommodation or gastric emptying in FD) and sensory (hypersensitivity to GI distension) function. These abnormalities have been associated with distinct symptom patterns, for example the association of hypersensitivity to gastric distension with epigastric pain in FD. Historically, emphasis on motor abnormalities shifted towards visceral hypersensitivity during the 1990s. However, recent evidence showed that at least in a subgroup of FGID patients, visceral hypersensitivity may be driven by psychological (and thus brain) mechanisms.

8.3.2 **Peripheral and central sensitization in FGID**

Peripheral sensitization (PS) is defined as the sensitization of peripheral primary GI afferent nerves. Inflammatory mediators (including histamine, bradykinin, prostaglandins and cytokines) reduce the transduction threshold of primary afferents and recruit previously 'silent' nociceptors, even in the absence of overt inflammation, by inducing expression of ion channels and receptors on nerve endings. This process may persist long after the insult, contributing to the GI hypersensitivity found in FGID patients. Primary visceral afferent neurons may contribute to GI pain hypersensitivity through the following mechanisms: (i) peripheral inflammation (ongoing cytokine expression in the absence of histological changes) (ii) visceral nerve damage (iii) changes in the number or function of several ion channels, initiated and maintained by presently unknown means. All of these potential mechanisms could result in visceral pain hypersensitivity without further amplification of visceral afferent input at CNS level. However, it is more likely that the peripheral input adds to the CNS mechanisms.

Sensitization of spinal cord dorsal horn neurons (amplified responses to both noxious and innocuous inputs, due to facilitated excitatory synaptic responses and depressed inhibition) is referred to as *central sensitization* (CS). Glutamate, together with other neurotransmitters such as tachykinins (substance P), plays a key role in this process. A human model demonstrated that infusion of hydrochloric acid into the healthy oesophagus reduced pain threshold not only in the acid-exposed region (PS) but also in the adjacent unexposed region (CS). This effect was prolonged and its duration and magnitude were related to the intensity of acid exposure. Repeated exposure after recovery significantly enhances the effect of the first infusion, suggesting that repeated injury can induce a progressive increase in hypersensitivity. Studies have also shown that central sensitization plays a role in IBS patients as well as patients with non-cardiac chest pain.

8.3.3 **Role of psychological factors in FGID**

Stress induction studies in healthy volunteers have shown that various forms of stress, including experimentally induced anxiety, influence gastric sensorimotor function including rectal and gastric compliance and gastric accommodation to a meal as well as symptom reporting.

Co-morbidity of FGID with psychiatric disorders (especially mood and anxiety disorders) is high, not only in treatment-seeking patients but also in community samples. We believe psychiatric co-morbidity should be assessed systematically in FGID patients and referral to mental health professionals with experience with functional somatic syndrome patients should be made if needed. This is especially important as evidence for a key role of psychological factors in generating GI hypersensitivity and symptoms in FGID is growing rapidly. Thus, at least in some patients, psychiatric disorders may not only be co-morbid, but may exert an important influence on the generation and reporting of GI symptoms.

The hypersensitivity to rectal distension observed in IBS patients may be at least partly attributable to hypervigilance towards visceral stimuli (a psychological tendency to report pain and urge) rather than increased neurosensory sensitivity. These findings are confirmed by cortical evoked potential research, which allows one to discriminate between afferent input and cognitive processing at the level of the brain. Furthermore, gastric sensory thresholds correlate negatively with anxiety scores in FD patients with hypersensitivity to gastric distension. An association between hypersensitivity to gastric distension and history of abuse, the personality trait neuroticism (characterized by a tendency towards negative affectivity) and somatization has also been found in FD.

Psychological factors including perceived stress, anxiety, somatization and negative illness beliefs have also been shown to predict the onset of IBS after acute gastroenteritis, which is consistent with the cognitive-behavioral model of IBS. This model is further supported by studies showing an association of depression and worrying with affective aspects of GI pain in IBS. This association was mediated via catastrophic thinking. Furthermore, 'gastrointestinal-specific anxiety' (defined as anxiety related to GI sensations, symptoms or the context in which these occur) has been shown to be a predictor of IBS status as well as a key mediator of the relationship between general psychological distress (including depression, anxiety) and IBS symptom severity. In FD, somatization and depression have been shown to be the strongest independent predictors of symptoms including pain, with gastric sensorimotor function not being an independent predictor.

8.3.4 **Functional brain imaging findings in FGID**

8.3.4.1 *Irritable Bowel Syndrome*

Generally, painful rectal distension activates similar brain regions in healthy volunteers and IBS patients (the 'visceral sensory neuromatrix'). However, patients and controls differ in terms of level and extent of activation, primarily in regions involved in the affective and cognitive aspects of GI pain. Some studies showed more ACC/MCC activity during rectal distension in IBS patients, compared to healthy volunteers. These differences may be explained by upregulation of visceral afferent input to the brain, abnormal affective or cognitive responses in the brain (increased anticipation, attention (hypervigilance) or negative affective reaction to the visceral sensory stimulus), or both. However, several other studies found less ACC/MCC activity in IBS patients. This can again be explained in different ways, including failure to activate descending antinociceptive pathways originating in the ACC/MCC, ceiling effects (with patients already being hypervigilant or anxious at baseline) or differential sensitization of the lateral versus the medial pain system in IBS.

Recent studies, including the first longitudinal brain imaging study in IBS, suggest similar afferent input to the brain in healthy controls and IBS patients when repeatedly exposed to rectal distension. Activity in an arousal/affective/ cognitive network, on the contrary, was higher in IBS patients and this hyperactivity normalized upon repeated exposure to the rectal distension stimulus, suggesting that IBS patients may be more vigilant and aroused when first studied, with habituation developing when studied repeatedly. This hyperactivity may also trigger the failure to activate descending antinociceptive pathways found in IBS patients. Although these studies provide interesting new insights in the putative role of psychological factors in IBS, differentiating between the role of heightened afferent input and the role of abnormal brain processing remains problematic.

8.3.4.2 *Functional dyspepsia*
FD patients, most of whom were hypersensitive to gastric distension, showed similar activation of the lateral pain system (SI/SII) compared to controls, but at significantly lower intragastric pressures and volumes, with similar pain scores. This activation at lower intensity of the peripheral stimulus may be the neurobiological substrate underlying visceral hypersensitivity, but does not necessarily indicate that only heightened afferent input, and not central cognitive or affective processes are involved. Furthermore, no activation of any cingulate subregion was found in FD patients, contrary to controls, which may again be explained in several ways (see above).

8.4 Treatment of gastrointestinal pain in FGID

8.4.1 Pharmacological treatments

8.4.1.1 *Antidepressants*
Tricyclic antidepressants (TCAs), especially desipramine and amitriptyline, are most frequently studied. They are mostly used in low doses to treat FGID symptoms without comorbid psychiatric disorders, although in FGID patients with co-morbid depression or anxiety higher doses should be used. TCAs have mainly been shown to have a beneficial effect on abdominal pain in IBS,

without clear evidence for improving global IBS symptoms. Their exact mechanism of action in treating GI pain remains unclear, although the serotonin (5HT) and/or noradrenaline reuptake inhibition (SNRI) (which is believed to be the mechanism underlying their antidepressant effect) is probably also important for the GI analgesic or anti-hyperalgesic effect. It remains a matter of debate whether antidepressants in FGID work peripherally or centrally and whether their effect on GI symptoms is primary or secondary to antidepressant or anxiolytic effects. The broad effects of TCAs on neurotransmitter physiology may cause side effects which are of relevance to GI symptoms, including constipation caused by anticholinergic effects. Newer antidepressants with an SNRI mechanism of action may have fewer side effects, making them promising treatments for FGID. Studies are however lacking and the use of duloxetine in FGID may be limited because of the frequently occurring nausea. Mirtazapine, a noradrenaline and selective serotonin antidepressant (and its older brother mianserin), may be promising in the treatment of FD, as it is lacking the GI side effects of the SNRI or SSRI antidepressants, but studies are currently not available.

Selective Serotonin Reuptake Inhibitors (SSRIs) have less frequently been studied compared to TCAs. Most studies show an effect on overall well-being and quality of life in IBS, but not on core GI symptoms including pain. A recent study however did show a beneficial effect on global IBS symptoms and abdominal pain with the SSRI citalopram, which was independent of its effect on anxiety, depression and somatization.

8.4.1.2 *Other agents*

Prokinetic agents, including D_2-antagonists (domperidone, metoclopramide) and $5HT_4$-agonists (tegaserod) have been used to treat FD (whether or not with delayed gastric emptying) and constipation-predominant IBS (showing improvement of global as well as individual IBS symptoms). Results of studies in FD have been mixed, and tegaserod has recently been withdrawn from the market due to (controversial) cardiac safety issues.

Fundus-relaxing drugs including the α_2-receptor agonist clonidine and the $5HT_1$-receptor agonist buspirone have been shown to improve symptoms associated with impaired gastric accommodation in FD, but only in small studies.

The *$5HT_3$-antagonist alosetron* significantly reduces global IBS symptoms in diarrhoea-predominant IBS, as it slows colonic transit but its use is also restricted due to—controversial—safety issues (risk of colonic ischaemia).

There is some, although not very strong, evidence for the effect of *antispasmodics, bulking agent laxatives and antidiarrhoeal agents* on abdominal pain, constipation and diarrhoea, respectively, in IBS.

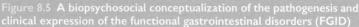

Figure 8.5 **A biopsychosocial conceptualization of the pathogenesis and clinical expression of the functional gastrointestinal disorders (FGID)**

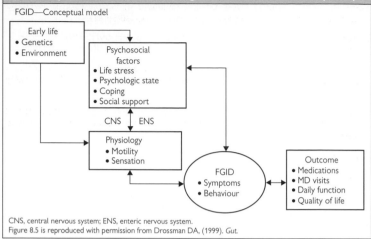

CNS, central nervous system; ENS, enteric nervous system.
Figure 8.5 is reproduced with permission from Drossman DA, (1999). *Gut.*

8.4.2 **Psychological treatments**

Hypnotherapy, various forms of psychotherapy [cognitive-behavioural therapy (CBT) as well as psychoanalytic interpersonal therapy] and, to a lesser extent, relaxation and biofeedback, have been shown to be cost-effective treatments in IBS, reducing abdominal pain as well as psychological distress, and to a lesser extent also in FD. A recent study showed that CBT has a direct effect on GI symptoms in IBS, independent of its effect on psychological distress.

8.5 **Conclusion**

Gastrointestinal pain in FGID is a biopsychosocial phenomenon resulting from a complex reciprocal interaction between biological (GI sensorimotor function), psychological (anxiety, …) and social (history of abuse, …) factors. The concept of the brain-gut axis allows us to understand this interaction (Figure 8.5). Treatment should therefore also be biopsychosocial in nature, with multidisciplinary care being the most promising.

Key references

Anand P, Aziz Q, Willert R, Van Oudenhove L (2007). Peripheral and central mechanisms of visceral sensitization in man. *Neurogastroenterol Motil.* **19**(1 Suppl): 29–46.

Aziz Q, Thompson D (1998). Brain-gut axis in health and disease. *Gastroenterology.* **114**(3): 559–78.

Clouse RE, Lustman PJ (2005). Use of psychopharmacological agents for functional gastrointestinal disorders. *Gut.* **54**(9): 1332–41.

Clouse R, Mayer E, Aziz Q, Drossman D, Dumitrascu D, Monnikes H, *et al.* (2006). Functional abdominal pain syndrome. *Gastroenterology.* **130**(5): 1492–7.

Drossman DA (2006). The functional gastrointestinal disorders and the Rome III process. *Gastroenterology.* **130**(5): 1377–90.

Jones MP, Dilley JB, Drossman D, Crowell MD (2006). Brain-gut connections in functional GI disorders: anatomic and physiologic relationships. *Neurogastroenterol Motil.* **18**(2): 91–103.

Lackner JM, Mesmer C, Morley S, Dowzer C, Hamilton S (2004). Psychological treatments for irritable bowel syndrome: a systematic review and meta-analysis. *J Consult Clin Psychol.* **72**(6): 1100–13.

Levy R, Olden K, Naliboff B, Bradley L, Francisconi C, Drossman D, *et al.* (2006). Psychosocial aspects of the functional gastrointestinal disorders.*Gastroenterology.* **130**(5): 1447–58.

Longstreth GF, Thompson WG, Chey WD, Houghton LA, Mearin F, Spiller RC (2006). Functional bowel disorders. *Gastroenterology.* **130**(5): 1480–91.

Moayyedi P, Soo S, Deeks J, Delaney B, Innes M, Forman D (2006). Pharmacological interventions for non-ulcer dyspepsia. *Cochrane Database Syst Rev.* **18**(4): CD001960.

Soo S, Moayyedi P, Deeks J, Delaney B, Lewis M, Forman D (2005). Psychological interventions for non-ulcer dyspepsia. *Cochrane Database Syst Rev.* **18**(2):CD002301.

Tack J, Bisschops R, Sarnelli G (2004). Pathophysiology and treatment of functional dyspepsia. *Gastroenterology.* **127**(4): 1239–55.

Tack J, Fried M, Houghton LA, Spicak J, Fisher G (2006). Systematic review: the efficacy of treatments for irritable bowel syndrome—a European perspective. *Aliment Pharmacol Ther.* **24**(2): 183–205.

Tack J, Talley NJ, Camilleri M, Holtmann G, Hu P, Malagelada JR, *et al.* (2006). Functional gastroduodenal disorders. *Gastroenterology.* **130**(5): 1466–79.

Van Oudenhove L, Coen SJ, Aziz Q (2007). Functional brain imaging of gastrointestinal sensation in health and disease.*World J Gastroenterol.* **13**(25): 3438–45.

Van Oudenhove L, Demyttenaere K, Tack J, Aziz Q (2004). Central nervous system involvement in functional gastrointestinal disorders. Best *Pract Res Clin Gastroenterol.* **18**(4): 663–80.

Chapter 9

Urogenital pain

Andrew Paul Baranowski

Key points

- Urogenital pain may be divided into the 'well defined' conditions and the Urogenital Pain Syndromes. For well defined pathologies the treatment of choice is the treatment of that pathology
- As well as pain, the Urogenital Pain syndromes will be associated with functional, sexual and psychological (cognitive, behavioural and emotional) symptoms
- Central nervous system sensitization changes, within the whole of the neuroaxis, may explain many of the pains, sensory dysphorias (such as urge to void) and functional changes
- Management of the Urogenital Pain Syndromes may involve treatments aimed at the specific syndrome. However, in many cases a generic symptomatic approach should be utilized. The tools available include—drugs, injections and neuro stimulation all aimed at neuromodulation, also psychological interventions and education/counselling.

9.1 Genitourinary pain

9.1.1 Background

The genitourinary system is a fusion between somatic and visceral systems with both systems being very specialized for their purpose and supported by a complex neuronal network. The somatic areas of the genitourinary system are particularly adapted for sexual activity and in particular sexual pleasure. This does raise some interesting questions about the neurological innervation of the urogenital system as a whole and as to whether the specialization seen within it (that produces the pleasant hyperaesthesia and orgasm of sex) contributes to produce the dysaesthesia and pain associated allodynia/hyperalgesia of some of the chronic pains associated with the vulva, clitoris and penis. Also, does this ability to undergo a physiological central sensitisation play a role in the deeper visceral associated pain syndromes?

9.1.2 **Classification and understanding the pain syndromes**

Over the past few years there has been a move towards separating out the 'well defined' classical pathologies that are associated with pain from the 'pain syndromes', where the pathologies are less well understood. 'Well defined' urogenital pathologies associated with pain would include: trauma, infection, inflammation, ischaemia, autoimmune disease, metabolic, cancer and structural problems associated with genetic and developmental disease. For the most part, management of the 'well defined' condition relies on management of the disease process in the first place and symptom management if primary treatment does not resolve the symptoms. It is not the remit of this chapter to discuss primary treatment of 'well defined' urogenital disease processes; however, it is important to emphasize the importance of diagnosing such pathologies and ensuring their appropriate management.

There are advantages and disadvantages of taking this dualistic approach, the main dilemma is—how and when do we decide to move on from investigating for a 'well defined' pathology? The European Association for the Study of Bladder Pain Syndrome/Interstitial Cystitis (ESSIC) have drawn up guidelines for the minimal investigations required to separate out the bladder 'confusable diseases' from the 'pain syndromes'. It is likely that other associations, including the European Association for Urology, Chronic Pelvic Pain, Guidelines Group (EAU CPPGG), will take a similar approach, developing diagnostic algorithms that then lead to treatment algorithms. It is interesting as to how ESSIC refer to 'confusable diseases' and not 'well defined pathologies'. This may reflect that pain in the urogenital system, for the main part, is not associated with a 'well recognised' pathological process and that for the main we should consider the 'pain syndromes'! Whatever the terminology, moving the process forward is important as the advantage of the dualistic approach is that once the decision has been made to move towards a pain syndrome diagnosis, management can become primarily symptomatic. An important part of this approach must be that a patient's diagnosis can change to become more appropriate as time progresses. The classification published by the EAU CPPGG recognized this and that general approach is becoming better accepted.

Once 'well defined' disease processes have been excluded and the diagnosis of a pain syndrome is made, the exact name of the syndrome will depend upon how confident the physician feels in being specific and is based on symptoms, signs and in some cases specific investigations. In general, most urogenital pain syndromes are considered as a part of the Chronic Pelvic Pain Syndromes; as the nature of the pain syndrome becomes clearer more specific diagnostic names can be given as one localizes the main site of perceived symptoms (Table 9.1).

Table 9.1 A classification approach for the Chronic Pelvic Pain Syndromes

Chronic pelvic pain (new definition)	Pelvic pain syndrome (1)	Urological	Painful bladder syndrome (1)	Interstitial cystitis	
			Urethral pain syndrome (1)		
			Penile pain syndrome (new definition)		
			Prostate pain syndrome (Adopted from NIH) (3)		
			Scrotal pain syndrome (1)	Testicular pain syndrome (new definition)	
				Post-vasectomy pain syndrome (new definition)	
				Epididymal pain syndrome (new definition)	
		Gynaecological	Endometriosis-associated pain syndrome (new definition)		
			Vaginal pain syndrome (1)		
			Vulvar pain syndrome (1)	Generalized vulvar pain syndrome (ISSVD 1999)	
				Localized vulvar pain syndrome (ISSVD 1999)	Vestibular pain syndrome (ISSVD 1999)
					Clitoral pain syndrome (ISSVD 1999)
		Anorectal	Proctalgia fugax (2)		
			Anorectal pain syndrome (new definition)		
			Anismus		
		Neurological	Pudendal pain syndrome (new definition)		
		Muscular	Perineal pain syndrome (1)		
			Pelvic floor muscle pain syndrome (new definition)		
	Well-defined conditions that produce pain, examples include:	Urological	Infective cystitis		
			Infective prostatitis		
			Infective urethritis		
			Infective epididymo-orchitis		
		Gynaecological	Endometriosis		
		Anorectal	Proctitis		
			Haemorrhoids		
			Anal fissure		
		Neurological	Pudendal neuropathy		
			Sacral spinal cord pathology		
		Other	Vascular		
			Cutaneous		
			Psychiatric		

85

Table 9.1 is modified from the EUA Chronic Pelvic Pain Guidelines (Fall RM, Baranowski AP, Elneil S, Engeler D, Hughes H, Messelink EJ, et al.; members of the European Association of Urology (EAU) Guidelines Office. Guidelines on Chronic Pelvic Pain. In: EAU Guidelines, edition presented at the 23rd EAU Annual Congress, Milan, 2008. ISBN 978-90-70244-91-0.
http://www.uroweb.org/nc/professional-resources/guidelines/online/)
Table 9.1 is reproduced from Fall M, Baranowski AP, Fowler CJ, et al. (2004). Guidelines on Chronic Pelvic pain. European Urology, 46(6): 681–9, with permission from Elsevier.

There are several important rules to this approach.

1. It is better to keep the diagnosis broad rather than to be too ambitious in ones presumptions, i.e. it is better to stay with Axis I rather than progress to Axis III in Table 9.1.

2. Symptoms may be localized in several organs within a system and even within several systems. A patient may thus have more than one syndrome. However, if a patient has multiple pain syndromes, it may be best to consider the patient under a broader term, i.e. it is better to stay with Axis I rather than progress to Axis III in Table 9.1.

3. Classifying the patient not only involves naming the syndrome, but should involve describing the symptoms—pain characteristics Axis IV, V and VI Table 9.1, as well as functional, sensory and psychological aspects, Axis VII and VIII Table 9.1.

4. Classifying a patient as suffering from a specific pain syndrome may open up avenues for specific treatments aimed at the specific pain syndrome. However, in the case of most patients, it is the symptoms that will need to be managed, hence the importance of Axis VII and VIII, Table 9.1.

Some examples of definitions are found in Table 9.2.

Table 9.2 Definitions used to describe the pelvic pains
Chronic pelvic pain is non-malignant pain perceived in structures related to the pelvis of either men or women. In the case of documented nociceptive pain that becomes chronic, the pain must have been continuous or recurrent for at least 6 months. If non-acute pain mechanisms are documented, then the pain may be regarded as chronic, irrespective of the time period. In all cases, there may be associated negative cognitive, behavioural and social consequences.
Pelvic pain syndrome is the occurrence of persistent or recurrent episodic pelvic pain associated with symptoms suggestive of lower urinary tract, sexual, bowel or gynaecological dysfunction. There is no proven infection or other obvious pathology
Scrotal pain syndrome is the occurrence of persistent or recurrent episodic scrotal pain that is associated with symptoms suggestive of urinary tract or sexual dysfunction. There is no proven epididymo-orchitis or other obvious pathology
Testicular pain syndrome is the occurrence of persistent or recurrent episodic pain localized to the testis on examination that is associated with symptoms suggestive of urinary tract or sexual dysfunction. There is no proven epididymo-orchitis or other obvious pathology
Epididymal pain syndrome is the occurrence of persistent or recurrent episodic pain localized to the epididymis on examination that is associated with symptoms suggestive of urinary tract or sexual dysfunction. There is no proven epididymo-orchitis or other obvious pathology

Table 9.2. This table illustrates some of the definitions used to describe the pelvic pains. A more in depth list can be found in the European Association for Urology Chronic Pelvic Pain Guidelines (Fall RM, Baranowski AP, Elneil S, Engeler D, Hughes H, Messelink EJ, et al. (2008).; members of the European Association of Urology (EAU) Guidelines Office. Guidelines on Chronic Pelvic Pain. In: EAU Guidelines, edition presented at the 23rd EAU Annual Congress, Milan, 2008. ISBN 978-90-70244-91-0. http://www.uroweb.org/nc/professional-resources/guidelines/online/).

Some of the definitions arise from the International Continence Society guidelines (Abrams P, et al., 2002) and further discussion is available in Urogenital Pain in Clinical Practice, edited by Baranowski AP, et al., 2007.

9.1.3 **The whole patient**

In a chapter on urogenital pain it is very easy to forget to consider the urogenital system as a whole and indeed that patients are persons. All conditions of the urogenital system, including the 'pain syndromes' are associated with a range of symptoms and signs which may be functional, sensory or psychological. Symptoms from all of these categories need to be addressed.

9.1.4 **Functional urogenital symptoms**

Functional symptoms may be associated with the primary problem or be secondary. Examples of functional problems associated with a primary condition would be: poor urinary flow and urinary frequency associated with prostatic cancer; infertility associated with infected pelvic inflammatory disease. Examples of secondary functional problems would be sexual difficulties, such as impotence associated with pain perceived within the testis; urinary frequency associated with urinary urge because of pain and urge to void perceived to arise from within the bladder but secondary to central neurological mechanisms. Secondary symptoms may require treatment in their own right. For instance, cGMP specific phosphodiesterase inhibitors for impotence secondary to pelvic pain or alpha 2 antagonists for poor urinary flow associated with the Prostate Pain Syndrome.

Functional symptoms do play an important part in how a patient is managed, as localized function syndromes lend to a belief that there is a local end organ pathology that requires some form of local intervention, such as surgery. However, the results of local procedures are poor. The reason for this is that in many cases the mechanism of the functional symptoms/signs overlaps with the sensory symptoms—that is, that they have a central neurological basis.

The central sensitisation changes well described in this book, as well as in other texts, will produce functional and sensory disturbance as well as pain. Afferent output as a result of the central changes that occur throughout the neuroaxis are a part of this. The functional symptoms may result from changes in afferent neurological control, changes in haemodynamic regulation, neurogenic oedema and/or smooth and/or striated muscle control. As examples, haemodynamic changes with plasma extravasation and neurogenic oedema may contribute to the haematuria found in certain patients with 'Haematuria Loin Pain Syndrome' or the glomerulations found in some patients with 'Bladder Pain Syndrome'.

9.1.5 **Muscle hyperalgesia**

The role of the striated muscles has been raised on many occasions. It is now well established that patients with pelvic floor muscle trigger points can complain of a range of pains and functional symptoms. The exact cause of such trigger points is not known; however, central sensitization is well established as a mechanism for muscle pain and hyperalgesia. Predisposing factors may include an acute stressful event (such as a negative sexual encounter, death of some one close to the patient, a life threatening incident), chronic stressful events (such as, difficult circumstances at work or within a relationship), or an acutely painful process (such as pelvic surgery, acute injury or acute genito urinary infection). Many patients in these circumstances will be aware of pelvic tension, but many will not. We all suffer from these symptoms to a certain extent—such as the pelvic discomfort and urge to void prior to an examination. In the pathological situation, on clinical examination trigger points within muscles will be discovered and should reproduce the patients' local pain as well as its radiation. Pelvic floor surface electromyograms may go some way to helping with the diagnosis. The functional symptoms associated with the muscle hyperalgesia may include: urinary hesitance, poor flow, frequency and urge in some cases of bladder base irritation. In other cases erectile, ejaculatory dysfunction and dyspareunia may be present. As well as being painful, the hyperalgesic muscles may produce secondary pain by nerve irritation (e.g., irritation of the pudendal, posterior femoral cutaneous nerve and sciatic nerves has been suggested) and by the mechanism of muscle induced central changes, musculovisceral hyperalgesias. It is because of the visceromuscular, viscerovisceral and musculovisceral induced hyperalgesias producing non-specific chronic pelvic pains that many experts wish to move away from the organ and system specific pain syndrome diagnostic approach and to use the more generic term of Pelvic Pain Syndrome.

9.1.6 **Sensory dysaesthesia**

As has been indicated, central changes within the neuroaxis may produce a pain syndrome. However, it has also to be appreciated that such changes can produce a whole range of sensory perceptions. As well as frank pain (often described in multiple terms), allodynia and hyperalgesia, other sensory symptoms exist—such as orgasmic sensations, itching, urge to urinate and with the bowel urge to evacuate. The debates about how these symptoms fit into a taxonomy are vociferous. For instance, does a patient with urinary urge (the sensation of needing to pass urine to reduce the sensation and not for fear of incontinence) suffer from a Bladder Pain Syndrome? A better understanding of the mechanisms may at some point help, but with the current understanding we remain unsure. As a consequence any decisions made now will have to be flexible.

9.1.7 **Nerve injury/irritation and pain perceived within the urogenital system**

There is no debate that nerve injury can produce pain and that pain is perceived in those areas innervated by the respective nerve. This is as true for the somatic nerves innervating the urogenital system as it is for any somatic area in the body. Recently, the importance of injury/irritation of the pudendal nerve has been raised as a cause of pain perceived in the anus, perineum, vulva and clitoris/penis. Pain from this nerve may also be perceived in the testis, bladder and deep within the pelvis. Other peripheral nerve pain syndromes causing loin pain, groin pain and buttock pain are well described. However, the question that remains is—what is the role of those afferents that travel within the autonomic pathways or indeed what is the involvement of the autonomics?

9.1.8 **Sexual dysfunction**

As with all chronic urogenital pains, the pain syndromes will be associated with sexual dysfunction and a matrix of psychological responses. Some of these sexual symptoms will be related to the central changes and may be functional. In many cases there may be a psychological underlying mechanism. Personal experience within our multidisciplinary urogenital pain clinic has taught me the complexity of these sexual symptoms, which are all too easy to ignore. The basis of their management has to be founded on a good understanding of what was normal for the patient and what is the normal range within the population. Advice should be non-judgemental, and should focus on non-painful sexual activity. A significant amount of time spent covering the sexual and relationship difficulties may be rewarded with a significant improvement in quality of life despite no change in the perception of pain.

9.1.9 **Psychological influences**

The psychological consequences of suffering from urogenital pain are not too dissimilar from those of other chronic pains. As for all chronic, persistent pains, the psychological response to the pain and the patient's innate psychological profile with its effect on the response to the pain need to be assessed and psychological interventions employed as appropriate. Urogenital pain experience will effect cognition, behaviour and emotion in negative ways. It is well established that catastrophizing, inappropriate pacing and maladaptive coping mechanisms in patients with chronic urogenital pain negatively influences the severity of pain significantly, reduces quality of life and increases disability (both sexual and general motor). As with any symptom, these need to be assessed and managed effectively as a part of our commitment to the care of the whole patient.

9.1.10 **The lack of a role for negative sexual encounters**

Negative sexual encounters have been a focus of contention in patients complaining of urogenital pain for many years. To date, the studies demonstrating a positive association between a history of negative sexual encounters in childhood and the development of chronic urogenital pain have been retrospective. There are considerable methodological problems in relying on retrospective report of childhood experience as abuse. The only prospective study on sexual abuse in childhood and subsequent development of pain in adulthood did not confirm that sexual abuse in childhood results in increased pain complaints in adulthood. It is accepted that severe sexual trauma at any age may produce long term structural and functional changes within the nervous system resulting in altered perception of pain. While the negative sexual encounter should be identified and managed as appropriate, in most cases it is inappropriate to label the patients as having a 'psychological' pain.

9.2 **The pain syndromes**

Table 1 places the pain syndromes into a structured classification. However, in view of the overlap of multiple mechanisms the specific syndrome approach has limitations and so specific treatments advocated for the pain syndromes (Table 9.3) must be considered in the context of the above explanation of the general mechanisms involved. As will be seen in Table 9.3, certain generic treatments aimed at the peripheral nerves, central sensitisation chronic pain mechanisms and their consequences of musculo- and viscero- hyperalgesia may be the way forward. Such treatments would include neuropathic analgesics and injection treatments. Injections aimed at specific nerve pathways may also have diagnostic value. There is significant evidence to support a psychological approach that will include cognitive behavioural therapy as well as other psychological techniques. It is rare that psychiatric techniques will have to be resorted to, though occasionally extreme depression, anxiety or persistent chronic illness behaviour resistant to psychological intervention may require psychiatric assessment.

Table 9.3 summarizes in an easy to read format the treatment options. A more in depth appraisal may be found in Baranowski *et al.*, 2007).

Table 9.3 **The evidence base behind some of the treatment options for some of the urogenital pain syndromes**		
Condition	Treatment	Level of evidence
Bladder Pain Syndrome/ Interstitial cystitis	Cimetidine	Ib
	Sodium pentosan polysulfate (oral and IV)	Ib
	Intravesicular Dimethyl Sulfoxide	Ib
	Amitriptyline	Ib
	Hydroxyzine	II
	Oxybutinin, gabapentin, bladder training, biofeedback	V, minimal but logical consideration
	Neuromodulation	III
	Cognitive behavioural therapy and other psychological approaches	Studies for chronic pain show excellent results, research for urogenital pain underway
Prostate Pain Syndrome (NIH III a or b prostatitis, prostadynia)	Diazepam, baclofen, tizanidine	II

Table 9.3 (Contd.)		
Condition	**Treatment**	**Level of evidence**
	Alfuzosin, tamulosin	II
	Cognitive behavioural therapy and other psychological approaches	Studies for chronic pain show excellent results, research for urogenital pain underway
	Antibiotics (if patient demonstrates a response)	II
	Analgesics	V, mainstay of treatment, but little evidence they improve quality of life
	Physiotherapy and biofeedback aimed at pelvic floor muscles	II
Renal Pain Syndrome	Treatment of overlying muscle hyperalgesia	V, minimal evidence but logical consideration
	Renal nerve blocks	III
	Cognitive behavioural therapy and other psychological approaches	III
Testicular Pain Syndrome	Local anaesthetic injections and L1 root nerve blocks	IV
	Surgery for discreet pathology, denervation and orchidectomy	III
	Antibiotics (if patient demonstrates a response)	III
Generic treatment options	Neuropathic analgesics, tricyclic antidepressants, anticonvulsants	Grade I for neuropathic pain
	Opioids	If a trial is successful and only if appropriate guidelines are followed (e.g., Recommendations for the appropriate use of opioids in persistent non-cancer pain (2005), The British Pain Society)
	Differential nerve blocks	III, may also have a role in diagnosis
	Trigger point therapy, manipulation, local and steroid injection, botulinum toxin	III/IV

Table 9.3. This table illustrates the evidence base behind some of the treatment options for some of the urogenital pain syndromes. The information is summarized by Baranowski AP from: Baranowski AP, Abrams P and Fall M (eds)(2007). Urogenital Pain in Clinical Practice, Taylor and Francis; Fall M, Baranowski AP, Elneil S, Engeler D, Hughes J, Messelink EJ, et al. (2008); members of the European Association of Urology (EAU) Guidelines Office. Guidelines on Chronic Pelvic Pain. In: EAU Guidelines, edition presented at the 23rd EAU Annual Congress, Milan, 2008. ISBN 978-90-70244-91-0. http://www.uroweb.org/nc/professional-resources/guidelines/online/; Hanno P (2005). Painful Bladder Syndrome (including interstitial cystitis). Committee. 21:1–66.

I Systematic review of all randomized controlled trials, II At least one randomized controlled trial, III-1 Well-designed, pseudo-randomized trial, III-2 Comparative study with a concurrent control group, III-3 Comparative study with a non-concurrent control group or two single-arm studies, IV Case series, V expert opinion.

Key references

Abrams P, Baranowski A, Berger RE, Fall M, Hanno P, Wesselmann U (2006). A new classification is needed for pelvic pain syndromes—are existing terminologies of spurious diagnostic authority bad for patients? *J Urol*. **175**(6): 1989–90.

Abrams P, Cardozo L, Fall M, Griffiths D, Rosier P, Ulmsten U, *et al.* (2002). The standardisation of terminology of lower urinary tract function: report from the Standardisation Sub-committee of the International Continence Society. *Neurourol Urodyn*. **21**(2): 167–78.

Anda RF, Felitti VJ, Bremner JD, Walker JD, Whitfield C, Perry BD, *et al.* (2006). The enduring effects of abuse and related adverse experiences in childhood. A convergence of evidence from neurobiology and epidemiology. *European Archives of Psychiatry and Clinical Neuroscience*. **256**(3): 174–86.

Anderson R, Wise D, Sawyer T, Chan C Integration of myofascial trigger point release and paradoxical relaxation training treatment of chronic pelvic pain in men. The *J Urol*. **174**(1): 155–60.

Baranowski AP, Abrams P, Fall M (eds). (2007). Urogenital Pain in Clinical Practice. Taylor and Francis, Abingdon.

Baranowski AP, Abrams P, Berger RE, Buffington CA, de C Williams AC, Hanno P, *et al.* (2008). Urogenital pain—time to accept a new approach to phenotyping and, as a consequence, management. *Eur Urol*. **53**(1): 33–6.

Bielefeldt K, Gebhart GF (2006). Visceral pain: basic mechanisms. In: SB McMahon, M Koltzenburg (eds). *Textbook of Pain*. 5th ed. Churchill Livingstone, New York, pp. 721–36.

Buffington CAT (2004). Comorbidity of Interstitial Cystitis with other *Unexplained Clinical Conditions. Journal of Urology*. **172**: 1242–8.

Fall M, Baranowski AP, Fowler CJ, Lepinard V, Malone-Lee JG, Messelink EJ, *et al.* (2004). European Association of Urology. EAU guidelines on chronic pelvic pain. *Eur Urol*. **46**(6): 681–9.

Fall M, Baranowski AP, Elneil S, Engeler D, Hughes J, Messelink EJ, *et al.* (2008). Guidelines on Chronic Pelvic Pain. In: European Association of Urology (EAU) Guidelines, edition presented at the 23rd EAU Annual Congress, Milan, 2008. ISBN 978-90-70244-91-0. http://www.uroweb.org/nc/professional-resources/guidelines/online/).

Glazer HI, Jantos MA, Hartmann EH, Swencionis C (1998). Electromyographic comparisons of the pelvic floor in women with dysesthetic vulvodynia and asymptomatic women. *J Reprod Med*. **43**: 959–62.

Hanno P (2005). Painful Bladder Syndrome (including interstitial cystitis). *Committee*. **21**: 1–66.

Merwe JP, Van de, Nordling J, Bouchelouche P, Bouchelouche K, Cervigni M, Daha LK, *et al.* (2008). Diagnostic criteria, classification and nomenclature for painful bladder syndrome/interstitial cystitis: ESSIC proposal. *Eur Urol*. **52**(1): 60–7.

Nickel JC, Tripp D, Teal V, Propert KJ, Burks D, Foster HE, *et al.* (2007). Interstitial Cystitis Collaborative Trials Group. Sexual function is a determinant of poor quality of life for women with treatment refractory interstitial cystitis. *J Urol*. **177**(5): 1832–6.

Nordling J, Anjum FH, Bade JJ, Bouchelouche K, Bouchelouche P, Cervigni M, et al. (2004). Primary evaluation of patients suspected of having interstitial cystitis (IC). Eur Urol. 45(5):662–9.

Novi JM, Jeronis S, Srinivas S, Srinivasan R, Morgan MA, Arya LA (2005). Risk of irritable bowel syndrome and depression in women with interstitial cystitis: a case-control study. J Urol. 174(3): 937–40.

Raphael KG, Widom CS, Lange G (2001). Childhood victimization and pain in adulthood: a prospective investigation. Pain. 92(1–2): 283–93.

Raphael KG (2005). Childhood abuse and pain in adulthood—More than a modest relationship? Clin J Pain. 21(5): 371–3.

Robert R, Labat JJ, Bensignor M, Glemain P, Deschamps C, Raoul S, et al. (2005). Decompression and Transposition of the Pudendal Nerve in Pudendal Neuralgia: A Randomized Controlled Trial and Long-Term Evaluation. Eur Urol. 47: 403–8.

Rothrock NE, Lutgendorf SK, Kreder KJ (2003). Coping strategies in patients with interstitial cystitis: relationships with quality of life and depression. J Urol. 169(1): 233–6.

Tripp DA, Nickel JC, Wang Y, Litwin MS, McNaughton-Collins M, Landis JR, et al. (2006). National Institutes of Health-Chronic Prostatitis Collaborative Research Network (NIH-CPCRN) Study Group. Catastrophizing and pain-contingent rest predict patient adjustment in men with chronic prostatitis/chronic pelvic pain syndrome. J Pain. 7(10):697–708.

Chapter 10

Visceral pain in cancer patients

Sebastiano Mercadante

Key points

- Visceral cancer pain originates from primary or secondary lesions involving hollow and parenchymal organs
- Visceral pain is poorly localized initially and often referred to distant somatic structures
- Most pain is responsive to systemic opioid analgesia
- Spinal analgesia should be considered after appropriate trials with systemic opioids
- Neurolytic sympathetic blocks can be helpful in decreasing opioid consumption.

10.1 Introduction

Visceral cancer pain is more frequently seen in patients with abdominal and pelvic tumours and originates from primary or metastatic lesions involving the hollow organs of gastrointestinal or genitourinary tracts and the parenchymal organs. Visceral cancer pain is often misconstrued as originating from somatic structures and is often referred to distant sites. The poor correlation between visceral injury and pain and the apparent insensitivity of some visceral organs have not been clearly elucidated. The late clinical presentation may be explained by the high threshold for painful stimuli, with a relative insensitivity of viscera, and the need for an adequate as well as specific stimulus. Initially, visceral pain is poorly localized and dull because of the wide divergence of visceral afferents in the spinal cord. Better localization of the stimulus occurs when the disease extends to a somatically innervated structure, such as the parietal peritoneum, due to sensitization of dorsal horn neurons sharing input from both visceral and somatic sites.

10.2 **Pain causes**

There are different causes of pain. Extensive intrahepatic metastases, or gross hepatomegaly associated with cholestasis, may produce discomfort in the right flank, due to distension of the capsule. Diaphragmatic irritation due to abdominal distension produced by large subdiaphragmatic masses may induce shoulder pain, and may be associated with hiccup. Pain may be exacerbated by movement or pressure and is frequently associated with nausea. Pancreatic cancer or retroperitoneal masses involving the upper abdomen may produce pain by infiltrating the coeliac plexus, local inflammation, and injury to vascular structures and is often associated with the involvement of deep somatic structures. Patients with abdominal or pelvic cancer may have abdominal pain due to chronic intestinal obstruction. Contributing factors include smooth muscle contractions, mesenteric traction, and mural ischemia. Both continuous and colicky pain are diffuse and often referred to dermatomes.

Cancers or radiotherapy in the pelvis produce progressive pelvic and perineal pain, as well as other complications, including ureteric obstruction and lymphatic and venous obstruction. Invasion of the tumour into the rectum or bladder can lead to erosion with bleeding sloughing of the tumour into the urine or bowel, and bladder or bowel obstruction. Renal colic is commonly secondary to ureteral obstruction and subsequent distension of the ureter and renal pelvis. This may be evident in circumstances in which an abdominal-pelvic mass compresses or invades ureters, as often occurs in gynecological cancers. Other causes of pain are often observed in pelvic cancers, due to the involvement of the ileopsoas muscle, lumbosacral plexus and presacral area, retroperitoneal spread, adding an important neuropathic pain component. In advanced disease, visceral malignancies spread to involve the somatic pleura or peritoneum, producing additional localized pain of somatic origin (Box 10.2).

10.3 **Pharmacological treatment**

Most pain in cancer responds to pharmacological management using orally administered analgesics. The current treatment approach is based on an analgesic ladder, which is essentially a framework of principles rather than a rigid protocol. When patients with cancer experience severe pain, opioids are

---

Box 10.1 Principal visceral syndromes associated with cancer

- Hepatic distension syndromes
- Midline retroperitoneal syndrome
- Chronic intestinal obstruction
- Peritoneal carcinomatosis
- Malignant perineal pain
- Ureteric obstruction.

the mainstay of therapy. There is a large variety of options for the delivery of opioids in the management of cancer pain. In some instances, there are clear indications for using one preparation or delivery system rather than another.

10.4 Around the clock analgesia

10.4.1 Non-opioid analgesics

NSAIDs have been claimed to have a major role in the management of some specific cancer pain syndromes, including pain from bone metastasis, soft-tissue infiltration, arthritis and recent surgery. In patients with cancer pain, NSAIDs are useful both for somatic and visceral pain as the first step of the analgesic ladder, also in combination with opioids, regardless of the pain mechanism involved. However, prolonged use should be discouraged, particularly in the elderly.

10.4.2 Opioids

Opioids are the mainstay of cancer pain treatment. The second step of the analgesic ladder, including opioids for moderate pain, such as codeine and tramadol, may be skipped by using adequate doses of strong opioids. Systemic opioids can be given by different routes. The oral route is the most common, least invasive, and easiest route for opioid administration for most patients with cancer pain, and morphine is the most popular drug. The doses are titrated against pain until dose stabilization is reached, resulting in adequate analgesia and acceptable adverse effects. Although dose titration with the immediate release preparation is recommended, it is desirable to use extended-release preparations to provide longer-lasting analgesia. If additional analgesia is needed for 'breakthrough' pain during dose titration, doses of a fast-onset, short-acting opioid preparation should be prescribed. Oxycodone, methadone, and hydromorphone are possible alternatives to oral morphine, no opioid being demonstrated to be superior to the other ones. Other options are represented by transdermal drugs. Many patients will develop tolerance to most of the undesirable side effects of opioids (such as nausea/vomiting or sedation) over a period of several days; therefore, a medication should not be labelled 'intolerable' until a reasonable trial has been undertaken. However, in the presence of persistent adverse effects, unresponsive to symptomatic drugs, opioid switching may be useful in improving the balance between analgesia and adverse effects, based on existing asymmetric tolerance among opioids. This may allow the use of lower doses than expected according to equivalency tables, with global improvement of the global opioid effects. Opioid conversion ratios for switching should be considered only as approximate indications (Table 10.1).

10.4.2.1 Alternative routes for opioid administration

Certain patients may not be able to ingest oral medications because of swallowing difficulties, gastrointestinal obstruction or nausea and vomiting. Alternative routes include the intravenous, subcutaneous and transdermal

Table 10.1 Approximate equivalence table for opioid conversion		
	Oral	**Parenteral (IV-SC)**
Morphine	60	20
Oxycodone	40	
Methadone	8–12	
Hydromorphone	8–12	
TTS fentanyl	12	
Buprenorphine	0.7	

ones. Various opioids are available for intravenous adminstration in the majority of countries, including morphine, hydromorphone, fentanyl and methadone. The oral-parenteral ratio for morphine is about 2.5:1. For patients requiring parenteral opioids who do not have in-dwelling intravenous access, the subcutaneous route can be used. This simple method of parenteral administration involves inserting a small plastic cannula on an area of the chest, abdomen, upper arms or thighs and attaching the tubing to an infusion pump. The main advantages of the subcutaneous over the intravenous route is that there is no need for vascular access, changing sites can be easily accomplished. For these reasons it fits home care and hospice setting.

For stable patients unable to take oral medications, the transdermal route is the preferable option for maintaining continuous plasma concentrations of opioids. Lipophilic and potent drugs have to be used for this modality of administration. Reservoir and, more recently, matrix systems have been developed to deliver a 3-day supply of fentanyl. Upon initial application of the patch, a subcutaneous 'depot' is formed as fentanyl saturates the subcutaneous fat beneath the patch. After approximately 12 hours, steady-state plasma fentanyl concentrations are reached, which are maintained for about 72 hours. Fentanyl patches are currently available in 25, 50, 75, and 100 microgram/hr (per BNF) dosages. Because of the slow depot formation and slow rise in plasma concentrations, this system is not suitable for rapid titration of pain and is best suited for patients with stable pain in whom the 24-hour opioid requirement has already been determined. Elevation of body temperature secondary to fever will increase blood flow to the skin and increase drug diffusion into the systemic circulation. Transdermal buprenorphine, delivered by a matrix system, is also available in releasing different dosages. Similarly to fentanyl, transdermal delivery of buprenorphine provides a slower increase in serum concentration and no peak-and-trough effects as seen with the sublingual route of administration. Although the use of this drug has been considered as problematic, because of the possible antagonist effect with other opioids, at clinical doses this is unlikely to occur and the global effect is compatible with an additive type of interaction.

10.4.3 **Breakthrough pain**

Breakthrough or episodic pain is a transitory flare of pain superimposed on an otherwise stable pain pattern in patients treated with opioids. A decrease in analgesia is observed in different situations, including end-of-dose failure, particularly during opioid titration, incident pain, for example due to movement in patients with bone metastases, or unknown causes. The availability of supplemental doses of opioids (rescue medication) in addition to the continuous analgesic medication is the main treatment suggested to manage these pain flares. Current dosing recommendations for breakthrough pain generally suggest that the effective dose of breakthrough pain medication must be a percentage of a patient's total daily opioid dose. However, an oral dose form can take a longer time to relieve pain. A short onset of effect is commonly obtainable only with parenteral or transmucosal administration of opioid analgesics.

Transmucosal administration of opioids is an attractive solution because it offers the potential for a more rapid absorption and onset of action relative to the oral route. Lipophilic drugs are better absorbed via this route than are hydrophilic drugs. Oral transmucosal fentanyl has been shown to be a safe and effective treatment for breakthrough pain and to have some advantages over oral opioids. Other preparations will soon be available (intranasal, inhalatory, sublingual).

10.5 **Spinal analgesia**

A small number of patients may still fail to obtain adequate analgesia despite large systemic opioid doses, or may suffer from uncontrollable side effects such as nausea, vomiting, or oversedation. These patients may be candidates for the administration of a combination of opioids, local anaesthetics, and clonidine via the spinal (epidural or intrathecal) route. Intrathecal opioid administration has the advantage of allowing a higher concentration of drug to be localized at the receptor site while minimizing systemic absorption, thus possibly decreasing drug-related side effects. Other advantages include the small volumes for pump recharge and fewer mechanical complications.

Morphine remains the drug of choice for the spinal route, because of its relatively low lipid solubility. It has a slow onset of action but a long duration of analgesia. The starting dose to calculate should take into consideration various factors, including the previous opioid dose, the age and the pain mechanism. Adding a local anesthetic (bupivacaine or ropivacaine) to morphine via the spinal route has been successful in providing good analgesia in patients whose pain was resistant to epidural morphine alone, despite high doses. Clonidine, α.-adrenergic agonist that acts at the dorsal horn of the spinal cord to produce analgesia. There is some evidence to suggest that neuropathic pain may be somewhat more responsive to the combination of clonidine/morphine than to morphine alone, although orthostatic hypotension is of concern. Procedural and surgical complications, system malfunction and pharmacological adverse effects are the main categories of complications associated with spinal drug delivery.

10.6 **Neural blockade**

In visceral pain sympathetic fibers are responsible for the transmission of noxious stimuli. Interruption of sympathetic pathways has been widely applied to relieve abdominal visceral pain. In comparison with somatic blocks, such as spinal neurolysis, burdened by severe neurological complications, sympathetic blocks have a low complication rate. The classic targets of sympatholysis in cancer pain are the coeliac plexus, the superior hypogastric plexus and ganglion impairment. Due to the frequent involvement of somatic structures or nerve injury, particularly in pelvic cancers, these blocks should be considered as adjuvants to opioid therapy.

10.6.1 **Coeliac plexus block**

Neurolytic coeliac plexus block (NCPB) is indicated for abdominal pain from cancers of the upper abdomen. Controlled randomized studies have reported prolonged efficacy of NCPB and the use of neurolytic agents may provide long-term relief that could match the life expectancy of cancer patients. Various techniques differing in terms of anatomical approach, solution injected, instruments used and radiologic guidance methods have been proposed in an attempt to improve the analgesic effects while avoiding complications. NCPB may offer other benefits in addition to analgesia, in part by decreasing the dose of opioids and a general increase in patient alertness. Suppression of sympathetic tone may also result in increased bowel motility with decreased constipation and less nausea with increased appetite.

Failure of the block may be attributable to concomitant pain of somatic origin, frequently observed in upper gastrointestinal cancer, due to large peritoneal involvement, requiring other therapeutic measures. Other causes of the failure of NCPB include technical problems, the presence of tumour in the area of the coeliac plexus preventing the spread of the neurolytic substance or the presence of metastases.

10.6.2 **Superior hypogastric block**

Superior hypogastric plexus block has been claimed to be highly effective to control pelvic pain syndromes. Clinical problems concerning neurolytic superior hypogastric block are nearly the same as for coeliac plexus block. Both control visceral pain. However, the less favourable results obtained with the hypogastric plexus block may be due to the greater tendency of pelvic tumour to infiltrate somatic structures and nerves compared to pancreatic tumour where the coeliac plexus block is usually used.

10.6.3 **Ganglion impar block**

Visceral pain in the perineal area associated with malignancies may be treated with neurolysis of the ganglion impar. This ganglion, located at the level of sacrococcygeal junction, marks the end of the two sympathetic chains. The possible candidates who can benefit from this block are patients presenting a vague and poorly localized pain, associated with burning sensation and urgency. Long-term data on the effectiveness of this block is, however, limited.

10.6.4 **Punctate midline myelotomy**

Recently, the dorsal column was revealed to play a more important role than the spinothalamic tract in visceral signal transmission. Punctate midline myelotomy (PMM) was introduced to treat intractable abdominal and pelvic pain in patients with advanced cancer. This approach has been described as having fewer neurological complications and proven efficacy in the treatment of otherwise intractable abdominal and pelvic cancer pain. As there are still no prospective randomized clinical trials, the argument for this technique is largely empiric. Among the concerns is that positive results will be easier to be published than negative ones. Moreover, even when clinical trials report positive outcomes, the long-term benefits of these treatments have not been sufficiently demonstrated. Finally, tumours invading the lumbosacral plexus and spine may generate new types of pain that are difficult to treat. Thus, PMM has still not found its place in the algorithm of clinical pain management.

10.7 **Conclusion**

The oral route of opioid delivery should be the first choice in the management of cancer pain, due to its simplicity, reproducible in any setting, particularly at home. Available opioids most commonly used are morphine, oxycodone, hydromorphone and methadone, as well as transdermal drugs, including fentanyl and buprepnorphine. For the treatment of breakthrough pain transmucosal fentanyl offers a more rapid effect in comparison with oral opioids. Opioid switching has been found to be effective to improve the opioid response. Non oral routes also include the intravenous or subcutaneous administration.

The intrathecal route should be started when multiple trial of systemic opioids have failed. This route may be most successful when opioids and local anaesthetics and/or clonidine are used in combination. Whatever route is used, administration of opioids to manage cancer pain requires knowledge of potency relative to morphine and bioavailability of the route chosen. Therefore, patients should be closely followed and doses titrated to minimize side effects whenever the opioid, route, or dose is changed. Neurolytic sympathetic blocks should be considered as an adjuvant treatment to reduce opioid consumption and opioid-related adverse effects, and not as a last resort, when the advantages of the blocks seem to be minimal.

Key references

Cervero F, Laird JMA (1999). Visceral pain. *Lancet.* **353**: 1245–48.

De Leon Casasola O (2000). Critical evaluation of chemical neurolysis of the sympathetic axis for cancer pain. *Cancer Control.* **2**: 1242–8.

Hong D, Andrén-Sandberg A (2007). Punctate midline myelotomy: a minimally invasive procedure for the treatment of pain in inextirpable abdominal and pelvic cancer. *J Pain Symptom Manage.* **33**: 99–109.

Hanks GW and the Expert Working group of the Research Network of the European Association for palliative care (2001). Morphine and alternative opioids in cancer pain: the EAPC recommendations. *Br J Cancer.* **84**: 587–93.

Mercadante S (1999). Opioid rotation in cancer pain: rationale and clinical aspects. *Cancer.* **86**: 1856–66.

Mercadante S, Radbruch L, Caraceni A, Cherny N, Kaasa S, Nauck F, *et al.* (2002). Steering Committee of the European Association for Palliative Care (EAPC) Research Network. Episodic (breakthrough) pain: consensus conference of an expert working group of the European Association for Palliative Care. *Cancer.* **94**(3): 832–9.

Mercadante S (1999). Problems of long-term spinal opioid treatment in advanced cancer patients. *Pain.* **79**: 1–13.

Mercadante S, Catala E, Arcuri E, Casuccio C (2003). Coeliac plexus block for pancreatic pain: factors influencing pain, symptoms and quality of life. *J Pain Symptom Manage.* **26**: 1140–7.

Regan JM, Peng P, Chan V (1999). Neurophysiology of cancer pain: from the laboratory to the clinic. *Curr Rev Pain.* **3**: 214–25.

Sevcik MA, Jonas BM, Lindsay TH, Halvorson KG, Ghilardi JR, Kuskowski MA, *et al.* (2006). Endogenous opioids inhibit early-stage pancreatic pain in a mouse model of pancreatic cancer. *Gastroenterology.* **131**(3): 900–910.

Skaer TL (2004). Practice guidelines for transdermal opioids in malignant pain. *Drugs.* **64**: 2629–38.

Index

103